D0108618

DATE DUE

Restoration of Normal Movement after Stroke

To Dr Beat Selz-Keller and his team in the neuro-rehabilitation unit at Bürgerspital, Solothurn, Switzerland, where the Johnstone concept is both practised and taught.

For Churchill Livingstone

Commissioning editor: Mary Law
Project editor: Dinah Thom
Project manager: Valerie Burgess
Project controller: Nicola Haig/Pat Miller
Copy editor: Teresa Brady
Indexer: Nina Boyd
Design direction: Judith Wright
Sales promotion executive: Maria O'Connor

Restoration of Normal Movement after Stroke

Margaret Johnstone FCSP
Private Practitioner, UK; Consultant Physiotherapist to Physiotherapie Institut, Bürgerspital, Solothurn, Switzerland; presently involved in clinical research, UK

Illustrated by
Estrid Barton

With an introduction by
James Cox MD FRCP (Edin, Lond)
Consultant Physician, Medicine for the Elderly and General Medicine, Cheviot and Wansbeck NHS Trust, Wansbeck Hospital, Northumberland, UK

CHURCHILL LIVINGSTONE
EDINBURGH HONG KONG LONDON MADRID MELBOURNE
NEW YORK AND TOKYO 1995

CHURCHILL LIVINGSTONE
Medical Division of Pearson Professional Limited

Distributed in the United States of America by Churchill Livingstone, 650 Avenue of the Americas, New York, N.Y. 10011, and by associated companies, branches and representatives throughout the world.

First published 1995

ISBN 0 443 052476

British Library Cataloguing in Publication Data
A catalogue record for this book is available from the British Library.

Library of Congress Cataloging in Publication Data
Johnstone, Margaret, FCSP.
Restoration of normal movement after stroke/Margaret Johnstone; illustrated by Estrid Barton.
p. cm.
Includes index.
ISBN 0–443–05247–6
1. Cerebrovascular disease--Patients--Rehabilitation. 2. Movement disorders--Patients--Rehabilitation. I. Title.
[DNLM: 1. Cerebrovascular Disorders--rehabilitation. 2. Rehabilitation--methods. WL 355 J73Ra 1995]
RC388. 5. J619 1995
616.8' 1--dc20
DNLM/DLC
for Library of Congress

94-41153
CIP

The publisher's policy is to use **paper manufactured from sustainable forests**

Produced by Longman Singapore Publishers (Pte) Ltd
Printed in Singapore

Contents

Preface

In recent years more and more of those who are involved in the rehabilitation of the stroke patient see a need for a team approach. Without the full co-operation of all those who care for these patients (whether this care is hospital or home based) and without a clear understanding of the physical disability that has overcome the individual patient, the rehabilitation programme will fail and the stroke victim will not be given a fair chance of realizing his or her full recovery potential.

Facing up to the physical problems caused by the brain damage of stroke is the concern of the rehabilitation team. Early in the treatment plan abnormal muscle tone has to be recognized. There is an urgent need to deal with the problems this presents and usually this involves addressing the ever increasing challenge of spasticity. However, normal movement depends on close interaction between motor and sensory events. The brain damage of stroke frequently results in sensory loss, and the problems posed by sensory loss must also be considered. For example, loss of proprioception may cause severe and persistent handicap. The undamaged brain receives information through a number of different sensory channels (proprioception, or the sense of muscle and joint position, being one of these) and this information is analysed by the central nervous system. Previous experience (memory) puts this information into context; it is processed in the brain which then responds, producing behaviour immediately appropriate for any environmental situation with the necessary motor responses. Sensorimotor integration is vital if the appropriate responses are to be made to achieve normal movement with postural adjustments as required. Sensorimotor systems have to initiate and coordinate all required movements for any situation while posture is dependent on a continuous flow of sensory information about events in the environment. Loss of the memory of normal movement readily becomes a major problem after the onset of a stroke if the damaged brain is allowed to accept the abnormal and often bizarre movements produced by released reflexes which now lack cortical control; it soon becomes a very difficult task to replace the memory of normal movement. If rehabilitation is to be effective, solutions must be found to take care of abnormal muscle tone, to establish ways and means of stepping up sensory input and to prevent the loss of the memory of normal movement.

The purpose of this book is to present rehabilitation principles which are aimed at overcoming these formidable barriers to recovery of normal function of muscles and movement in the stroke patient.

Thirty years of work carried out with patient participation in the clinical field, searching for answers to the rehabilitation problems, is now well behind me and this book is based on that clinical search. Neurological facts suggested practical answers; or, sometimes, the discovery of a technique which repeatedly worked to good effect led back to the examination of established neurological facts, to find out why a specific technique gave a valuable contribution to recovery.

Throughout these years of discovery I met and was guided by other workers facing the same concerns. Some of them have been acknowledged in the text of the book, but there are others who have not been mentioned. I am indebted to Ann Thorp, my sister and fellow physiotherapist, who has travelled with me to many parts of the world, helping to turn our teaching courses into successful joint presentations. I also gratefully acknowledge the deeper understanding I have gathered from lectures I have attended given by neurological teachers, in particular in Switzerland by Professor Dr H-R Luscher of Berne and Professor Dr H P Clamann also of Berne. Both came on two different occasions to give an in-depth input to the teaching courses we presented in Switzerland at Solothurn, organized there by Dr Beat Selz-Keller of the Medizinische Klinik Bürgerspital, Solothurn. He travelled from Switzerland some 13 years ago to study for himself the rehabilitation method I use in clinical practice where there is neurological damage, and to assess my rehabilitation results.

Since then he and his physiotherapy staff, in particular Gail Cox Steck, have given me dedicated and constant support in my work and we have established a neurological rehabilitation centre with his leadership at Solothurn. We are spreading from there, sending out Accredited Teachers in the Johnstone concept who have come from other countries to study the Johnstone method. This is an encouraging beginning. Dr Selz holds the central register of Accredited Teachers at Solothurn. So far this includes teachers in Belgium, New Zealand, Switzerland, Britain, Germany and America and includes physio- and occupational therapists. To maintain a sufficiently high standard of practice, this certificate is not awarded unless candidates spend a certain amount of time at Solothurn, where they must prove their ability to practise and teach the rehabilitation principles and techniques involved in this approach to physical recovery.

I would also like to mention with particular thanks the help and support given to me by Rosemary Lane FCSP, formerly Principal of the Aberdeen School of Physiotherapy, and her invaluable teaching on tonal balance and reflex activity which led to my greater understanding of the stroke patient's needs.

Going back to my early days some years after I qualified, I have to acknowledge my thorough grounding in proprioceptive neuromuscular facilitation (PNF) as presented by the late Dena Gardiner. My 5-week training course with her made rehabilitation come alive for me and, in the following years, because of my understanding of PNF principles and techniques, I believe I became a better clinician.

I am also grateful to all the patients who have contributed to my understanding and have so cheerfully cooperated with me in the clinical field.

Since developing the rehabilitation programme presented in this book, Ann Thorp and I have, over the last 10 years, continued to use pressure techniques in the clinical setting and have widened our horizons considerably to include, for example, insult to the brain in road traffic accidents. With Ann Thorp's previous considerable clinical experience in neurological rehabilitation, particularly with multiple sclerosis patients, we have developed therapeutic inflatable splints as distinct from the URIAS stroke series. We have also become interested in cerebral palsy and have developed a third series of smaller splints for children of all ages. We gratefully acknowledge the help given to us by Claus Gerlöv Jeppesen of URIAS splints, Denmark. Users' guides for these splints are available from the distributors. These splints add a new and exciting dimension to rehabilitation.

For the sake of clarity, throughout the text of this book, the patient is referred to as 'he' and the therapist, nurse, helper or family member as 'she'.

Edinburgh 1995 M. J.

INTRODUCTION

J. Cox

SOME ASPECTS OF MEDICAL STROKE MANAGEMENT

To many physicians in the past, physiotherapy was all that could be offered to the stroke patient, and stroke care was almost always characterized by a lack of medical interest. This introduction provides a selective view of the current medical perspective and practical issues involved. As the majority of strokes (70–80%) are caused by cerebral infarction (Fig. i), the discussion will be concerned with cerebral infarction unless stated otherwise. The patient on the ward who has a hemiparesis is the most obvious sufferer from stroke, but medical attention should address wider issues. First, it is important to prevent stroke.

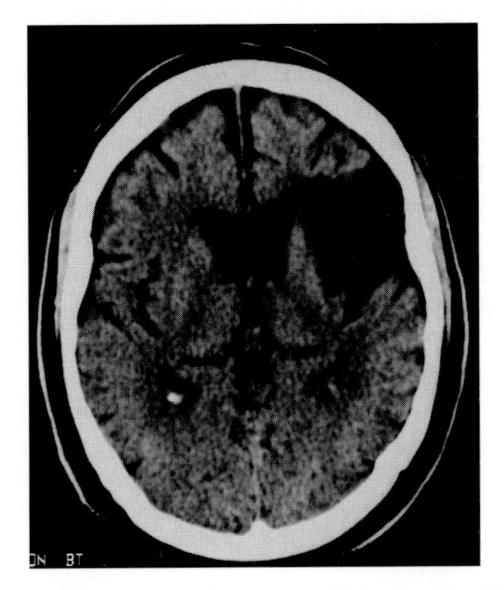

Fig. i Non-contrast cranial CT scan showing an established cerebral infarction (wedge-shaped dark area).

PRIMARY PREVENTION

The prevention of a stroke in a previously fit person is called primary prevention. This is carried out by general practitioners, who identify patients with the following modifiable risk factors for stroke:

- hypertension
- atrial fibrillation
- diabetes
- cigarette smoking
- heavy alcohol consumption
- drug abuse.

Treatment of these factors can reduce the risk of stroke. Hypertension is an obvious example of such a risk factor. Another example is non-rheumatic atrial fibrillation; several trials have shown that warfarin given to sufferers reduces the risk of stroke by two-thirds. The use of warfarin may also be economical if control is good, saving the taxpayer a potential £70 million per year – money that could be spent on other aspects of health care. Strategies to select subgroups of patients with atrial fibrillation who gain particular benefit from warfarin may lead to the greatest health and economic benefits.

Good health education, which emphasizes the importance of blood pressure control and the avoidance of cigarettes, is helpful. The greater awareness of the public about stroke, its prevention and in due course its treatment should also influence the incidence and effect of stroke. Governments should promote public awareness and also ban cigarette advertizing.

Primary prevention can help those at risk only if they are identified. Screening through well man/woman clinics identifies those with hypertension and these who smoke. Computerization in the surgery allows general practitioners to call up and target patients known to have other risk factors as new developments occur. Without computerized registers to identify the patients with known atrial fibrillation, the results of the research on warfarin for atrial fibrillation could not have been exploited. New ideas, such as open access echocardiography to look for cardiac abnormalities, may extend the role of screening by general practitioners for selected patients with known cardiac abnormalities, such as murmurs or atrial fibrillation. Studies to assess the benefit of screening selected patients with no previously known cardiac abnormality for atrial fibrillation are in progress.

Hypercholesterolaemia has not been proven to cause cerebral infarction, and the risk associated with the combined oral contraceptive pill appears to be very small. Although a heavy alcohol consumption may predispose to stroke, a mild to moderate alcohol intake reduces the risk of stroke.

If a patient has a transient ischaemic attack (TIA) or minor stroke, further strokes may be prevented if a cause is found. This is called secondary prevention.

THE ACUTE STROKE

Despite primary prevention, stroke is still common. What can be done for those who suffer acute cerebral infarction?

Diagnosis

The diagnosis of acute cerebral infarction has in the past usually been a clinical one in the UK because of the lack of computed tomography (CT) scanners. A clinical diagnosis and a 'wait and see' policy was thought reasonable in view of the lack of treatments both for stroke and its future prevention. However, as therapy for prevention is now available for some stroke patients and treatment soon may be, the use of CT scanning in the diagnosis of stroke is increasing. The initial objective is to diagnose, by CT, whether the stroke is due to infarction or to haemorrhage. After a diagnosis of cerebral infarction has been made, the physician should analyse why it occurred.

Medical treatment

Despite a great deal of recent research, there is no current proven treatment for patients with acute cerebral infarction. The best hope at present is that early thrombolysis to dissolve the intra-arterial clot may repeat the success that has seen in acute myocardial infarction. This is the subject of major international trials and some answers should be available in 1995. If the treatment works, it will be a major breakthrough in the treatment of acute stroke and will have considerable implications for the management of the stroke patient. For example, patients would have to be fast-tracked to and in the hospital in the same way as patients with myocardial infarction. Before treatment, an urgent CT scan would be necessary to exclude a cerebral haemorrhage. As up to 30% of patients with acute stroke in the UK are managed at home at present, the availability of treatment would increase hospital admissions as well as, hopefully, reducing disability and length of stay. All this will have an impact on professionals' and the public's attitudes to stroke and the resources needed for stroke patients.

It is unlikely that one kind of treatment alone will be effective in aborting all cerebral infarctions. Current research into the mechanisms of stroke and drugs to treat stroke or limit its damage include studies of calcium antagonists and high dose heparin. There are also studies into free radicals, which are compounds which are formed after a stroke and which may contribute to the death of neurones. Drugs which interfere with this process may have potential to limit stroke damage.

Surgical treatment

In my opinion, there is little place for surgery in management of acute cerebral infarction. However, occasionally a patient with a cerebral haemorrhage may benefit from surgery in the acute phase. This is usually when a patient with a posterior fossa haemorrhage develops rapid onset hydrocephalus and becomes drowsy. There is a risk of coning from raised intracranial pressure and urgent surgery to evacuate the clot may be life saving.

The multidisciplinary team

The best sort of care for stroke patients can be given only if the professionals involved work as a team. Those professionals who work in isolation may mar the final outcome for the patient. The contribution of skilled nursing in the management of the acute stroke patient is not emphasized enough. Good nursing with appropriate technology will help to prevent painful shoulders and pressure sores. Correct positioning, specialized lifting techniques and high quality alternating pressure mattresses are all important. The nurses are also responsible for early and repeated ward assessment of swallowing and, with the consultant, play a major role in liaison with relatives. A physiotherapist can spend only so much time with each patient and that is usually during the week. As the nurses spend longer with the patient, common aims are essential. In our unit, multidisciplinary team working is routine; the nurses, speech and occupational therapists and physiotherapists work together. It is important that all the nurses who lift or place the patients are educated in the appropriate techniques. Early involvement of the care manager is wise for appropriate discharge planning. I believe the concept of team working is just as important for physicians to grasp as it is for the nurses or therapists.

The physician's role

It is up to the physician to make the diagnosis, assess its severity and likely prognosis and then set it in the context of the patient's general health and likely aspirations. It is wise to discuss the diagnosis personally with the family to establish the reliability of the history and background information, to communicate what one can of the likely prognosis and to start a liaison with them for future planning.

Many studies have tried to predict the likely outcome for a stroke patient. The difficulties are numerous as the variability of patients, their previous illnesses and disabilities, the type, size and site of the stroke, the presence of an ischaemic penumbra (see below), and the attitude and aspirations of patients and relatives do not all fit into tidy protocols. Despite the difficulties, the Bamford classification (Table 1) is a simple and useful tool for subdividing cerebral infarction on clinical findings and can be used by the multidisciplinary team to discuss prognosis and progress.

Table 1 The Bamford classification of stroke

TACI Total anterior cerebral infarction
Motor and sensory deficit
Ipsilateral hemianopia
New disturbance of higher cerebral function

PACI Partial anterior cerebral infarction
Any two of the above
or isolated disturbance of higher cerebral function

POCI Posterior circulation infarct
Unequivocal signs of brainstem disturbance
or isolated hemianopia

LACI Lacunar infarction
Pure motor stroke
or pure sensory stroke
or pure sensorimotor stroke
or ataxic hemiparesis

Classification is based on clinical findings at the time of maximal deficit from a single stroke.

Rehabilitation

Rehabilitation is the restoration of as much normal function as possible and is a process of continuous reassessment and appropriate goal setting. It is much easier if communication is good and the family knows what to expect and understands what is being done. Rehabilitation needs to be practical. Not all patients can perceive our rehabilitation goals or achieve them. It is important to make sure that discomfort is treated by positioning or analgesia. A patient in pain will be unhappy and will find it difficult to concentrate on rehabilitation. Some patients suffer profound loss of privacy and dignity after a stroke. For example, unless he is handled with sympathy and understanding, the patient who is incontinent in front of others in the physiotherapy department may decide never to return. Each patient should be treated as an individual.

Weekend visits home should be conducted as soon as possible to maintain morale. Sometimes one should forget 'dogma' and make early use of wheelchairs for very disabled patients, especially if they are getting disheartened by their lack of mobility and their level of dependence. If the patient is not getting anywhere, step back and think again, perhaps laterally: are your goals the same as the patient's and is rehabilitation leading where the patient wants to go? A positive attitude, perception, gentle handling and kindness are all essential.

Discharge home should be preceded by a multidisciplinary home visit and further discussion between the patient, the carers and the physician about risks and how to reduce them, and an appropriate follow-up plan or support programme.

PREVENTION OF COMPLICATIONS

Aspiration pneumonia and swallowing problems

Swallowing problems are common. From the moment the patient arrives on the ward it is wise to be watchful for aspiration. The traditionally performed gag reflex is of little use in assessing safe swallowing. All our patients are assessed on arrival by nurses who have been trained by speech therapists. This ensures that patients with swallowing problems are detected early. No patient with stroke is fed until he has been assessed. Both nurses and speech therapists should continue to reassess, as some patients develop cerebral oedema after admission and their swallowing deteriorates even if initially satisfactory.

The time taken for swallowing to recover is often surprisingly long, and it seems unfair to burden the patient with drips or nasogastric tubes for longer than is absolutely necessary. In our series of 75 consecutive patients with moderate to severe swallowing problems, the median length of time from stroke to full oral feeding was 88 days (the range was 24–413 days). I try not to use nasogastric tubes unless there is no alternative, because of the disadvantages: patient discomfort, the inconvenience of repeated insertions and the potential need for prolonged feeding. My personal policy is to advocate insertion of percutaneous endoscopic gastrostomy (PEG) tubes in appropriate patients if there are no signs of imminent recovery of swallowing at 7–10 days after stroke. This allows the patient to be free of troublesome drips, permits more therapy, and the patient and staff can be happy that his nutritional needs are being met.

Deep vein thrombosis and pulmonary embolism

Deep vein thrombosis (DVT) occurs in about 50% of patients with a hemiparesis. Prevention is desirable as pulmonary embolism may occurs and can be fatal. However, the incidence of pulmonary embolism is said to be less than 10% and the incidence of death from pulmonary emboli is low at less than 2%. If low dose heparin is to be given, the usual advice is that a CT scan must be performed to exclude a cerebral haemorrhage; unfortunately, CT scanners are still not available in many hospitals in the UK. Moreover, even if a scan excludes a haemorrhage and the stroke is due to an infarct, there is still the concern that haemorrhagic transformation of the infarct may be induced by heparin, making the risk of heparin exceed its possible benefit. More research is needed, therefore, to define the safest course to protect patients against DVT. At present physicians tend to divide themselves into two camps, namely the purists, who avoid heparin, and the rest, who give it sometimes without scanning. The answer to this controversy may be available in 1995 when the International Stroke Trial reports. In the meantime, a recent study of general surgical patients showed that TED stockings reduced the risk of DVT in surgical patients by 70% and it may be reasonable to consider their use rather than heparin for the stroke patient.

SECONDARY PREVENTION

Many stroke patients progress well and the aim then is to prevent further cerebral infarction by means of secondary prevention. Any 'stroke episode' that lasts less than 24 hours is a transient ischaemic attack (TIA). A TIA usually lasts minutes or even seconds. TIAs are a strong predictor of future stroke and for practical and research purposes are usually grouped with minor strokes lasting, for example, a few days before the return to normality. A previously fit patient who suffers either a TIA or a minor stroke is usually a particularly appropriate candidate for assessment for treatable causes of stroke before further infarction occurs. However, every stroke patient should be considered on his own merits.

How much is or can be done varies a great deal, depending on where the patient is and what is available locally. Many TIA patients do not consult their doctor; this could be improved by better patient education. Many general practitioners and consultants in the past have treated stroke and TIA patients with aspirin, without investigation. I believe that all affected patients should be considered for an initial investigation by their general practitioner and should then be referred, if appropriate, for a consultant's opinion. The ideal consultant service to the general practitioner and his patient is offered through a well organized, rapid access stroke/TIA clinic, where patients can be assessed and investigated with appropriate non-invasive technology, and where advice about future management can be given.

A minor stroke or TIA is an opportunity to emphasize the modification of the major risk factors; the patient should again be advised not to smoke and the blood pressure should be controlled. It is also an opportunity to identify whether the patient has carotid artery disease, cardiac disease, or perhaps a rarer treatable cause of stroke. The additional risk factors to be assessed in secondary prevention are as follows:

- carotid stenosis
- cardiac disease with intracardiac clot
- polycythaemia
- temporal arteritis, polymyalgia, polyarteritis and other cerebral vasculitides
- migraine
- syphilis (in high risk groups at least).

CAROTID ARTERY DISEASE

A carotid stenosis is usually indicated by the presence of a bruit heard over the carotid artery bifurcation, which is just below the angle of the jaw, although unfortunately not all carotid stenoses cause bruits. Carotid ultrasound is a very sensitive means of detecting a stenosis and can demonstrate its severity. The treatment of carotid artery disease depends initially on the degree of stenosis. There have been two major trials, one in Europe and another in North America, which showed that if the stenosis is less than 30% the best course is aspirin, that if the stenosis is over 70% the patient should be considered for surgical correction of the stenosis (carotid endartectomy) and that those with stenoses of 30–69% must await further studies but take aspirin in the meantime.

Why aspirin? The reason is that stroke or TIA in patients with carotid artery disease is frequently due to the adhesion of platelets into a clump at the level of the stenosis, which then embolizes to the head: aspirin reduces platelet stickiness and so prevents emboli. Treatment with aspirin is, overall, very safe despite the risk of gastrointestinal side-effects.

For those in the severe stenosis group, surgery may be indicated. However, this cannot be performed without a preliminary carotid angiogram to define the anatomy. The risk of the angiogram causing a disabling stroke is 1–5%; this is lower than the risk presented by leaving a critical stenosis alone but is high enough to emphasize the importance of having experienced radiologists and discussing the risks with the patient first. Moreover, in these studies the surgery was carried out in 'centres of excellence' and it may be difficult to achieve comparable results elsewhere until more surgeons become experienced in the technique. The overall morbidity and mortality rate is about 6%, and this figure would be much higher in frail patients with multiple pathologies. Preoperative selection is therefore very important: for many patients, surgery may be inappropriate or too dangerous. If a centre has a combined risk of angiography and surgery of greater than 10% then no overall benefit is likely to be gained from surgery.

What are the other alternatives? Carotid angioplasty, the dilatation of a carotid stenosis by a balloon catheter, sounds a very attractive alternative to surgery but it is still being evaluated, and studies comparing it with carotid surgery are in progress. Ticlopidine is another antiplatelet agent and may be more effective than aspirin, but it has troublesome side-effects (neutropenia). Other agents are awaited.

We do not yet know how to treat patients who are found to have asymptomatic carotid stenoses; more research is needed.

HEART DISEASE

Assessment of the heart after a stroke or TIA can be profitable for the patient: if a source of intracardiac clot is found, this can lead to treatment with warfarin to prevent embolization. A well-recognized source occurs in patients with rheumatic mitral stenosis. These patients are usually in atrial fibrillation and have large left atria: clots form inside and then embolize. There is no doubt about the benefit of warfarin in such patients. If the cardiac signs are difficult to elicit, echocardiography can confirm the diagnosis. Elderly patients with hitherto unrecognized rheumatic heart disease still present with stroke even though rheumatic fever itself is now rare, as many of them had mild childhood attacks and develop problems only in old age.

Far commoner, however, are patients with non-rheumatic atrial fibrillation, and these patients have been shown in a 1993 European study to have a greatly reduced risk of stroke if given warfarin: the risk is reduced from 12% to 4% per year. If warfarin cannot be given then aspirin should be considered, though this is less effective in this situation. Cardiac assessment can lead to the diagnosis of these major cardiac risk factors for embolic TIA or stroke:

- mitral stenosis
- atrial fibrillation
- recent anteroseptal myocardial infarction
- left ventricular aneurysm
- dilated cardiomyopathy
- bacterial endocarditis
- atrial myxoma.

If no clinical or laboratory abnormality is found to account for a TIA, giving aspirin seems to be a reasonable policy. Unfortunately, some patients do not receive prior warning of a TIA, or even if they do and are treated, they still progress to acute stroke.

AREAS OF PARTICULAR INTEREST

Treatment of hypertension after stroke

Blood pressure often rises after stroke and it is not yet known when to intervene. The concern is that lowering the blood pressure too quickly or too much may make matters worse by reducing cerebral perfusion and causing an extension of the stroke. Most physicians take a conservative course and introduce drugs if hypertension continues after a couple of weeks.

The ischaemic penumbra

This is the area round a cerebral infarct which is poorly perfused but has a potential for recovery. As it is dependent on good perfusion, it is vulnerable to over-treatment of hypertension. It may also be threatened by uncontrolled atrial fibrillation or polycythaemia, both of which may reduce cerebral perfusion. It may lead to difficulty in assessing prognosis: if the area is large then until perfusion improves the stroke may seem worse than it is, leading to an unduly poor prognosis.

Lacunar infarctions

These are small cerebral infarctions usually in the white rather than the grey matter. Many are due not to carotid or cardiac disease but to 'sludging' or so-called 'in situ thrombosis'. Longstanding hypertension seems to predispose to lacunar infarctions, which are of interest, firstly because magnetic resonance imaging (MRI) scanning has demonstrated them to be more common than previously thought (there may not be a history of a stroke episode), and secondly because their prevention and treatment are likely to be different than in a case of embolic cerebral infarction.

SUMMARY

1. Prevent stroke by screening and good health education (primary prevention).
2. Investigate patients with TIA/minor stroke for a treatable cause (secondary prevention).
3. Once stroke has occurred, rehabilitate with a multidisciplinary team.
4. Do not feed patients by mouth until assessed for swallowing ability, and continue to monitor swallowing carefully if the patient deteriorates.
5. Aim to prevent DVT with, at least, TED stockings.
6. Monitor progress carefully and give the patient and relatives realistic goals.
7. Await with interest the conclusions of the 1995 International Stroke Trial.
8. Conduct further research, especially large controlled trials, into better treatments.

Endpiece

If ultimately the patient fails to improve despite all the efforts and technology, remember this:

> *Guerir quelquefois, soulager souvent, consoler toujours.*
> *(To heal sometimes, to relieve often but to comfort always.)*
>
> (Anon, 15th century or earlier).

FURTHER READING

Bamford J 1991 Is it a stroke and what sort of stroke is it? Hospital Update: 890–899

European Atrial Fibrillation Trial Study Group (EAFT) 1993 Secondary prevention in non-rheumatic atrial fibrillation after transient ischaemic attack in minor stroke. Lancet 342: 1255–1262

European Carotid Surgery Trialists Collaboration Group 1991 MRC European carotid surgery trial: interim results for symptomatic patients with severe (70–90%) or with mild (0–29%) carotid stenosis. Lancet 337: 1235–1243

Fisher M, Bogousslavsky J (eds) 1993 Current review of cerebrovascular disease. Current Medicine

International Stroke Trial (IST), Neurosciences Trials Unit, University of Edinburgh, Edinburgh

Marshall R S, Mohr J P 1993 Current management of ischaemic stroke. Journal of Neurology, Neurosurgery and Psychiatry 56: 6–16

Mulley G 1985 Practical management of stroke. Croom Helm, London

North American Symptomatic Carotid Endartectomy Trial Collaborators 1991 Beneficial effect of carotid endartectomy in symptomatic patients with high grade carotid stenosis. New England Journal of Medicine 325: 445–453

Warlow C, Wade D, Sandercock P, Muir J, House A, Bamford J, Anderson R, Allen C 1987 Strokes. MTP Press, Lancaster

1
BUILDING ON EXPERIENCE

INTRODUCTION

A rehabilitation concept for the stroke patient, if it is to be taken seriously, should present a method which is eclectic, soundly based on neurophysiological principles taken from different sources, and tested and tried in the clinical field and only adopted if found to be useful and to give consistently satisfactory results. 'Treat what you find' is a succinct and valid maxim, as long as the treatment is based on proven neurological facts. Any worthwhile concept concerned with stroke rehabilitation is usually built on clinical experience and not solely on classroom theory.

This means that the rehabilitation physiotherapist must be well versed in neurology, and able to apply this knowledge in the clinical field to address the problems presented. She must be able to decide the aim of the treatment offered and, knowing the aim and the neurological background, should present techniques which will give every patient a chance of fulfilling his maximum recovery potential.

The practical therapy approach presented in this book is based on sound neurological facts and on a long clinical trial which has given consistently satisfactory results. The validity of any rehabilitation concept for the treatment of stroke must be judged by the results obtained. So, at the start of the long clinical trial, there were questions which had to be asked and answers which had to be found. The end result was a rehabilitation method concerned with muscles and movement and the restoration of normal movement.

The brain is a jigsaw which has been shattered and the pieces have to be reassembled. It should be noted that the residual damage varies from patient to patient; different and varied disabilities are to be found, but dealing first with the neurological damage which disrupts the normal function of muscle and movement will give the recuperating brain a stable base on which to reorganize and build recovery. The techniques presented in this book lead towards the required foundation.

THE AIM AND PURPOSE OF THERAPY

It is necessary to be quite clear about the primary aim of any therapy which is to be offered in the early days after the onset of a stroke. The aim and purpose of any worthwhile ongoing therapy programme is to be found by considering the neurological basis of loss of normal movement.

The aim is to give back to the brain-damaged patient inhibitory control over abnormal patterns of movement.

The purpose is to restore postural control.

MUSCLE TONE AFTER A STROKE

A 'hands-on' approach can very quickly establish that muscle tone is no longer normal. Concerning normal muscle tone the relevant points to note are that:

1. it is balanced
2. it is reflex in character, based on the reflex arc
3. it is more marked in the antigravity muscles.

These three facts immediately shed light on the abnormal tonal patterns that are to be found in post-stroke disability. Expensive equipment is not needed for the study and assessment of tonal patterns. A physiotherapist at the end of training can make an accurate assessment using a hands-on approach.

Immediately after the onset of a stroke, in the majority of cases, abnormal tone presents as hypotonus, or flaccidity, but very soon afterwards hypertonus, or spasticity, usually develops, and the spasticity patterns are set by antigravity muscles. Further examination frequently reveals loss of normal sensation and in a small percentage of cases the initial hypotonus persists.

The latest neurological teaching and neuroscientific studies concern the need of the brain to reorganize its function after a stroke, but this does not dispense with the urgent need for therapists and nurses to take care of the tonal imbalance and, where possible, sensory loss, so that recovery may have a sound foundation. Furthermore, this urgent need must be addressed in the early days after the onset of the stroke if patients are to be given a fair chance of a satisfactory recovery, with a return to normal movement.

In the attempt to find answers to the problems concerned with altered muscle tone and loss of normal movement, it is logical to apply classroom neurology (Cash 1977) and to adopt practices which have given results and to discard those which have not, beginning in this way to build on successful techniques and to develop a programme for recovery.

To start at the beginning, knowledge of the properties of normal muscle tone leads to understanding the functions missing after stroke, and suggests ways of dealing with the resulting abnormal tone.

1. NORMAL MUSCLE TONE IS BALANCED

This does not need complicated neurological explanation, but a simple consideration of the normal relationship between the flexors and extensors of any joint. It is useful here to consider the elbow in preference to any other joint because, in stroke rehabilitation, a return to normal movement of the elbow often poses one of the most difficult problems. The muscles concerned are *biceps* and *triceps*, reciprocally acting muscles, agonist and antagonist. To extend the elbow, triceps must contract and, as it contracts, biceps must relax if the elbow joint is to extend. So far so good, but why does this reciprocal innervation not occur after the brain damage of stroke? This leads to point 2.

2. NORMAL MUSCLE TONE IS BASED ON THE REFLEX ARC

The reflex arc is the basic functional unit of the nervous system. Again neurologists have made this easy for us to understand. As already stated, to extend the elbow triceps must contract and, as it contracts, biceps must relax. A signal from the brain activates motoneurones in the spinal cord (Fig. 1), triceps contracts and the elbow extends. However this cannot happen unless biceps lengthens, or stretches, and this does not happen in the stroke patient. Normally biceps also initially contracts to resist the opposing contraction of triceps. This is known as the stretch reflex, which in normal muscle tone acts to maintain body posture and opposing movement. In normal muscle action this stretch reflex, relayed to biceps, has to be inhibited if normal movement is to take place. This leads to the conclusion that there has to be some form of inhibition between reciprocally acting muscles (Fig. 1).

Inhibitory interneurones in the spinal cord play a crucial role in sequential movement (Miller & Einon 1980). Study Figure 1 again: there is an inhibitory interneurone between triceps motoneurone and biceps motoneurone and this inhibitory motoneurone also receives descending inputs from the brain, via the corticospinal tract. Stroke damage takes place in the brain, not in the spinal cord, so any upset in the normal maintenance of balanced tone must come from the brain, suggesting that in the stroke patient this reciprocal inhibition, or balance of muscle tone, has been disrupted by brain damage. The long experience of clinical assessment of many patients with marked spasticity of hemiplegic arms, has seemed to indicate that in all cases biceps was continuously contracting, making movement very difficult if not impossible. In recent years leading neurologists have been able to measure the electrical activity of muscles, and have demonstrated that post-stroke excitation of antagonist antigravity muscles is continuous where spasticity is a problem. Here, excitation of biceps has become continuous and so, with the stretch reflex no longer under inhibitory control, normal movement about the elbow

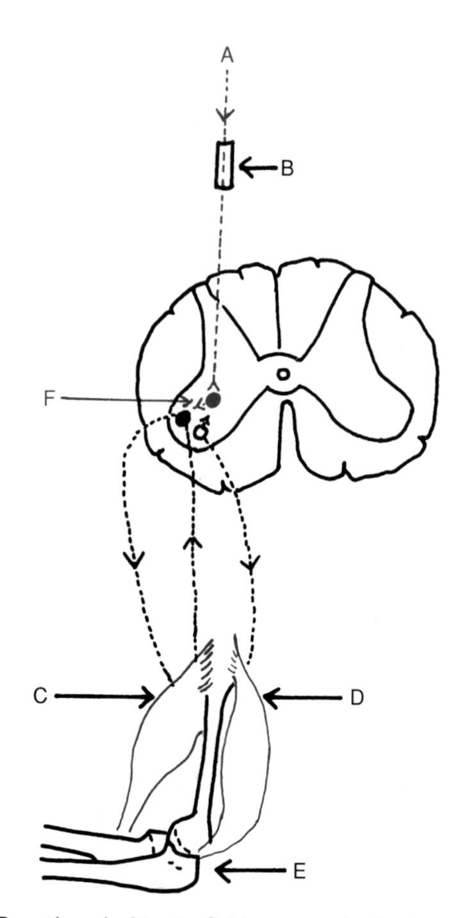

Fig. 1 A, brain input; B, corticospinal tracts; C, biceps muscle; D, triceps muscle; E, elbow joint; F, inhibitory interneurone.

joint is not possible. In the face of this, can the rehabilitation therapist find satisfactory answers to the problems presented?

3. NORMAL MUSCLE TONE IS MORE MARKED IN THE ANTIGRAVITY MUSCLES

This being the case, and with the opposing muscle groups out of balance because of lost inhibition from the brain to the stretch reflex, the consequent loss of the necessary reciprocal inhibition will result in severe residual problems.

For many years solving problems of this kind has been left to the physiotherapist. A possible answer can only be found if a satisfactory way of inhibiting the strong antigravity tone can be introduced. This inhibition would of necessity have to be offered by the environment, i.e. by forces outside the body. These would have to control and correct the patient's imbalance of muscle tone while rehabilitation is undertaken and reflex activity once more brought under cortical control. Can the therapist really make an effective contribution towards inhibiting the antigravity tone?

For a long time, an attempt has been made to do this by using inhibiting movement patterns and by lying, sitting and standing using inhibiting positioning at all times (Bobath 1970). However, although this line of thought and specialized treatment makes very sound sense, when offered, it is usually too little and too late. Nor can one therapist and one patient go it alone! In many cases strong antigravity patterns have taken over and the patient has become a helpless prisoner held fast in the crippling patterns of spasticity with no chance of regaining normal movement. The urgent need is to start the treatment *early* after the onset of the stroke and to *inhibit 24 hours a day.* Late treatment to reverse deformities that have developed usually takes a very long time with results that may be poor at best.

For the stroke patient to attain optimal recovery it is increasingly obvious that successful exercise programmes must concentrate on control of muscle tone, and of tonal flow, throughout the whole body while a reasoned and progressing exercise scheme is implemented. All the professionals involved, i.e. physiotherapists, occupational therapists, speech therapists, nurses and doctors should understand the neurological needs of the patient, and the reasoning behind the requirement for meticulous positioning in all treatment sessions and between treatment sessions. Where possible it is of great value if a family member or a concerned carer can be integrated into this team.

SENSORIMOTOR PROBLEMS

As if the above seemingly difficult task were not enough, there are other problems. Normal movement depends on close interaction between sensory and motor events and, almost always, with stroke patients one is faced with the problems presented by sensory loss. So, this seems even more to be a no-win situation, and patients and their caring back-up team, hospital- or home-based, become increasingly depressed with the lack of success in rehabilitation.

The central nervous system (the brain and spinal cord) receives information through a number of sensory channels (pathways). Previous experience (memory) puts this information into context. It is processed in the brain, which then responds by stimulating the necessary motor responses for behaviour immediately appropriate for any environmental situation.

Sensorimotor integration is vital for making the appropriate responses for normal movement, with postural adjustments as required. Sensorimotor systems have to initiate and coordinate all required movements for any situation, and so we understand that the control of movement and posture is dependent on a continuous flow of sensory information about events in the environment (Adams 1974).

Consider, for example, loss of sensory information in systems such as proprioception, vision, hearing and so on. This is one point which some therapists do not consider and yet it is of the utmost importance for successful rehabilitation. The loss of the memory of normal movement probably occurs very quickly after brain damage from stroke and, if the brain is allowed to accept the abnormal and often bizarre movements produced by the released reflexes, it soon becomes a very difficult task to restore the memory of normal movement.

To concentrate on one of the serious post-stroke failures in the sensory systems it is useful, particularly from the physical therapist's point of view, to study proprioception and what happens where it is lacking. Proprioception is the sense of musclar position or of muscle and joint position. When all the necessary information from proprioceptors is not reaching the sensory cortex due to brain damage, this loss may lead to disturbance of body image, i.e. the ability to feel a limb, to appreciate its place in space and its relationship to the body. Tactile sensation may also be impaired, or lack of coordination of sensory input may disturb perception of the spatial relationships of objects outside the body. It must be a demoralizing or totally devastating experience for a patient to be no longer aware of his body image and incapable of determining his position in space. Visual agnosia must also be recognized, but as a perceptual problem and not as blindness.

When considering proprioceptors, which are situated in muscles, tendons and joints, and their part in sensory integration, the role of the specialized proprioceptors which lie at musculotendinous junctions must also be examined. These are the Golgi tendon organs; they are receptive to sustained stretch and are known to have an inhibitory influence on motoneurone pools of their own muscle supply, that is, an autogenic effect (Cash 1974). Any reaction to sustained stretch in the treatment of stroke should be considered when attempting to restore reciprocal inhibition. So the question arises, is there a place for sustained stretch in the treatment of stroke and, if so, how may this be applied in the rehabilitation of stroke disability?

It becomes increasingly clear that answers must be found to all these questions. And there is another severe problem that has to be faced: what is to be done to control associated reactions (see below).

ASSOCIATED REACTIONS

It is also necessary to consider the associated reactions which are very much involved in the rehabilitation of the stroke patient. 'Associated reactions' are released postural reactions, deprived of voluntary control because of cortical damage. They occur with all attempted movements, to give a widespread increase of spasticity. They play a large part in the often all-too-rapid onset of spasticity in the weeks following a stroke and this, in turn, leads to a serious build-up of residual disability.

This prompts other questions to which rehabilitation therapists are expected to find an answer, namely: is there an effective way to divert these wayward reactions into inhibiting patterns? Or, is the use of inhibiting positioning enough or is some more dynamic form of treatment needed?

Strokes generally result from cerebral thrombosis, haemorrhage or embolism and, as already mentioned, they most usually have an initial stage of hypotonicity, or flaccidity, which rapidly develops into hypertonicity, or spasticity.

However, this is not always so, and therapists may be faced with the difficult task of rehabilitating flaccid limbs. Contributing factors to hypotonicity may be associated with cerebral shock, defective afferent information and sensory interruption. Additionally from careful assessment in the clinical field over many years, this seems to be frequently found where proprioceptive sense is deficient in left-sided disability. Proprioceptive loss in right-sided disability does not seem to produce a severely flaccid limb to the same extent, but this would be a question to be addressed by more research. However, for many years rehabilitation therapists have been left to find the answers to problems arising from prolonged hypotonicity and it has not always been possible to do this. It has to be remembered that this is a problem of the central nervous system rather than a peripheral one, arising from the brain damage of stroke, which affects normal function at spinal cord level.

Where sensory interpretation is deficient, there is a wide range of assessment tests that may be used to uncover areas of hidden mental damage. Deficit may be found in one or more areas, for example, in intellect, proprioception, communication, perception and so on, and difficulties are often hidden by the patient and will cause him great mental distress. For instance, physiotherapists and occupational therapists may not be aware of some of the hidden difficulties in communication and here the speech therapist is very much needed. It is a relatively easy task to see the patterns of spasticity and, with hands on the patient, to assess his tonal state and tonal flow as movement takes place. However, sensory deficit cannot be seen or felt by therapists. All therapists should be able to carry out thorough assessment tests and should be able to interpret the test results accurately.

THE POSTURAL REFLEX MECHANISM

There is also proven neurological information which has a bearing on the logical and reasoned planning of a sound rehabilitation programme.

Consider, for instance, the postural reflex mechanism. This depends on:

1. normal postural tone
2. normal reciprocal innervation
3. normal patterns of movement.

With postural tone no longer normal, reciprocal innervation out of gear and normal patterns of movement disrupted, there are obvious and severe problems that must be faced in making a useful approach to meaningful rehabilitation. The difficulty lies in how to do this and, at the same time, to deal with other motor problems, such as control of associated reactions. It would also be useful if, at the same time, dynamic sensory input could be offered.

Each neurological fact seems to present therapists with more rehabilitation problems which may be the outcome of neurological damage to the brain resulting from cerebrovascular accidents. The clear aim and purpose of the therapist are as stated earlier (p. 2). The student of neurology may be in danger of becoming too deeply involved in his subject, and finding himself trapped in a vicious circle from which he can see no way out, if he cannot apply basic neurological information concerning postural control to meaningful patient care. However, by taking the basic proven neurological facts one at a time, and by building on these, a relatively simple rehabilitation pattern emerges which frequently leads to highly satisfactory results.

If normal muscle tone and postural control can be restored, then the other reorganization needs of the brain will be given a firm foundation on which to build. This book is concerned with the restoration of motor function after stroke. To concentrate too early in the rehabilitation programme on the more obscure needs of reorganizing and restoring total brain function is to put the cart before the horse, and usually leads to very poor rehabilitation outcome.

A REHABILITATION CONCEPT DEALING WITH MUSCLES AND MOVEMENT

The rehabilitation concept presented in this book deals with muscles and movement. It does not set out to address all the many problems (e.g. cognitive difficulties) that may be found after stroke. It is an approach for dealing with the physically disabled victim, and goes straight to the heart of the matter: to reverse the hemiplegia by restoring normal muscle tone and normal sensory input, and to return the victim of this catastrophe to normal physical ability. Carefully applied while observing strict rules, in many cases it will succeed, providing a firm base for the full recovery programme. Developmental progressions are used, or a neurodevelopmental sequence, and to attempt to deal with perceptual problems, for example, without this solid foundation is to jeopardize rehabilitation recovery.

One point in particular, from a recent review on neuroplasticity (Stephenson 1993), should be noted and applied in the early days of treatment.

> *Latent areas of the brain can specialise to replace lost function and new pathways can form to by-pass the effects of lesions. However to achieve this successfully, intensive, repeated stimulation is required to place demands on the reorganising systems.*

The constant repetition of any one exercise has been a rehabilitation rule for many years but it is too often forgotten or ignored. Little or no recovery progress has been seen in rehabilitation where this rule is ignored. In long trials in the clinical field Johnstone techniques have been found to provide the solid base for structural reorganization of the damaged brain.

SUMMARY

To sum up, consider abnormal muscle tone first. With the loss of the necessary inhibitory input from the brain (Fig. 2) because of the brain damage of stroke, postural tone is no longer under control in relation to gravitational forces, and spasticity patterns are seen to follow antigravity patterns. Where hyper-

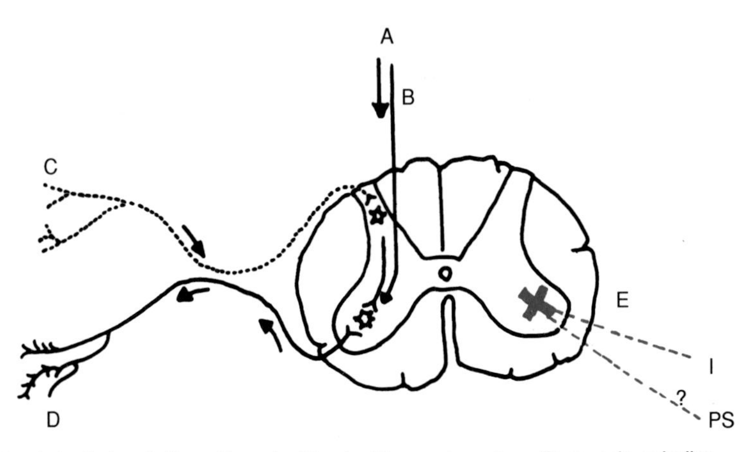

Fig. 2 A, brain input; B, corticospinal tracts; C, proprioceptors; D, muscle spindle; E, anterior horn. Major barriers to successful motor recovery: I, loss of inhibitory input from the brain; PS, loss of proprioceptive sense.

tonicity does not seem to be the problem and patients present with the 'floppy doll' limbs of flaccidity, or hypotonicity, eventually spasticity will usually also develop and may be noticed first in the fingers (Johnstone 1989).

Motor mechanisms are intimately related to, and functionally dependent on, sensory information. Or, to put it another way, normal movement depends on close interaction between sensory and motor events. So, with a lack of inhibitory output from the brain, and disruption of the necessary sensory input to the brain, the stroke patient is in serious trouble. In particular, where therapists are dealing with muscles and movement in an attempt to restore physical recovery, if proprioceptive sense is deficient, this major barrier to rehabilitation must be recognized and measures must be taken to increase sensory input. The question is, what can be done for there to be any chance of successful rehabilitation?

Figure 2 represents the major barriers to recovery of normal movement in the stroke patient. Common sense would suggest starting at spinal level and looking for a way round the obstacles, remembering the missing function which has caused the problems, and finding a way forward which will recover this missing function.

REFERENCES

Adams G F 1974 Cerebrovascular disability and the ageing brain. Churchill Livingstone, Edinburgh

Bobath B 1970 Adult hemiplegia: evaluation and treatment. William Heinemann, London

Cash J (ed) 1977 Neurology for physiotherapists, 2nd edn. Faber and Faber, London

Johnstone M 1989 Current advances in the use of pressure splints in the management of adult hemiplegia. Physiotherapy 75: 7

Miller S, Einon G 1980 Biology, brain and behaviour. Mechanism of muscle control – moving muscles. Open University course

Stephenson R 1993 Some implications for physiotherapy in the treatment of lesions of the brain. Physiotherapy 79: 10

2
START WITH THE TRUNK

Starting at spinal level, as shown in Figure 2, there is lost function between the damaged brain and inhibitory interneurones in the spinal cord, and also loss of proprioceptive sense. These are the two major rehabilitation problems that should be faced *early* in the recovery programme and satisfactory solutions must be found, otherwise physical recovery will fail.

Professor Norman Dott was an early pioneer in the difficult area of rehabilitation after severe brain damage. In the early days, because of the Second World War, patients with gunshot wounds of the brain came under his expert care. Many of these patients presented with spasticity problems and often with hemiplegia. Norman Dott, in his wartime unit in Bangour Village as Director of Neurology and Neurological Surgery, taught the therapists, including myself, who worked in his specialized unit to use neurodevelopmental exercise patterns (Hendrie & Macleod 1991).

From Bangour I moved into orthopaedics but, some years later when I took charge in an acute general hospital, I found myself faced with a constant stream of stroke patients. Little had been published on stroke rehabilitation. The practice at the time was to clamp the hemiplegic leg in a rigid metal caliper, and I felt this could not be right. Remembering Norman Dott's teaching I discarded the rigid caliper and set out to use developmental patterns. So, almost by accident, I began to build on experience in the clinical field. This led to a rehabilitation programme designed to meet the problems which were encountered and which would give a high standard of recovery.

The first tenet of this programme recognizes that one cannot build stability of the limbs on an unstable trunk.

Rule 1: Start with the trunk.

THE NORMAL DEVELOPMENT OF CONTROLLED MOVEMENT

Motor development in the infant is from head to foot in direction, that is from proximal to distal, or neck and shoulder before arm and hand, trunk and hip before knee and foot. Fetal movements are reflex movements and are called primitive, but it must be remembered that these primitive reflex movements are the predecessors of all purposeful, coordinated actions.

At birth, the first movements are all primitive; eye movements, head turning, kicking, finger grasp and so on. Most of us have watched these restless, primitive movements of the newborn child and, later, as the infant grows and the development of motor function goes forward, we have seen these primitive movements develop into controlled movement which can be performed deliberately or automatically. We have been watching the infant develop his postural reflex mechanism.

The infant learns to roll. Rolling is a new movement. He repeats it again and again as if he is practising his new trick; as, indeed, he is. With the constant repetition of this new movement, and because of the alterations of the position of his head in space and in relation to his trunk and extremities, postural and righting reflexes are called into action. Soon, rolling from supine to prone becomes a controlled and functional movement, and he rolls to prop on his forearms or he rolls into sitting, with the development of more complicated equilibrium responses.

He extends his head in prone and he crawls on his forearms dragging his legs. Forearm crawling leads to pushing himself backward and he gets onto all fours. Supporting himself in this position, he pushes himself backwards and forwards over his hands, freeing his primitive flexor grasp and releasing his hands for functional movement.

Postural stability and controlled movements progress: he pulls himself up onto his feet, he bears weight, shifts his weight, transfers from foot to foot, develops postural stability, the primitive movements of flexion and extension are modified and he walks.

This fascinating sequence of motor development can be followed in any healthy infant from birth through the early months of life. It is the outward and visible sign of inward and invisible reflex action, controlled movement and postural stability, developing concurrently with the nervous system. From intensive repetition of primitive movements which gain a reflex response he has developed controlled movement. Figures 3 and 4 represent some of the

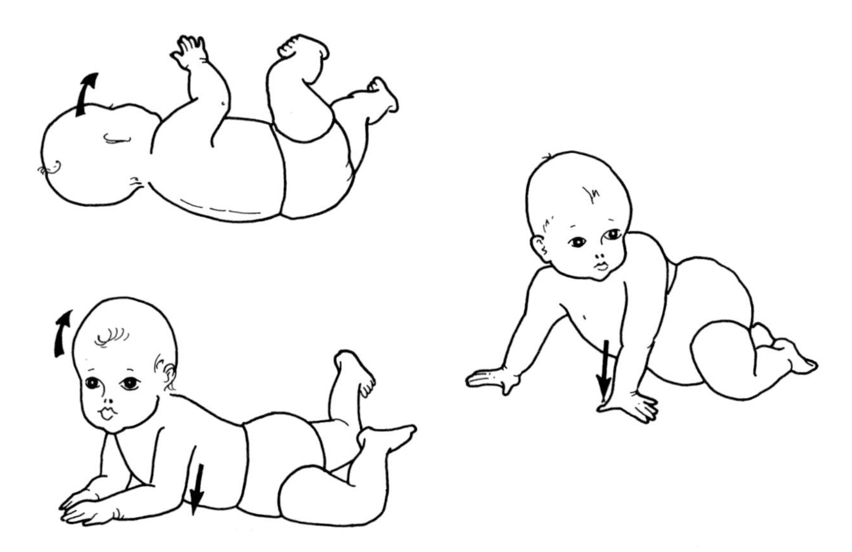

Fig. 3 Neuromotor patterns (1).

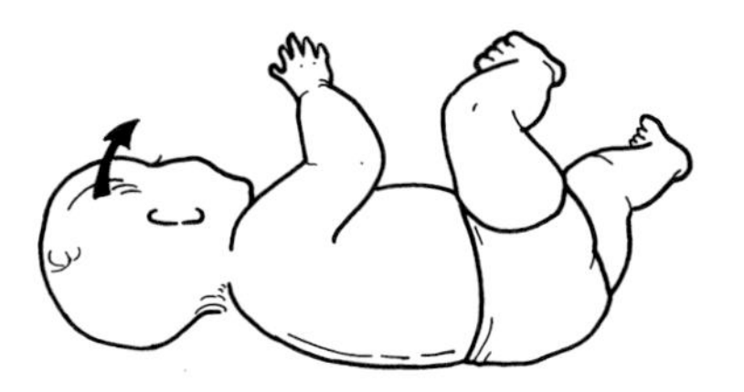

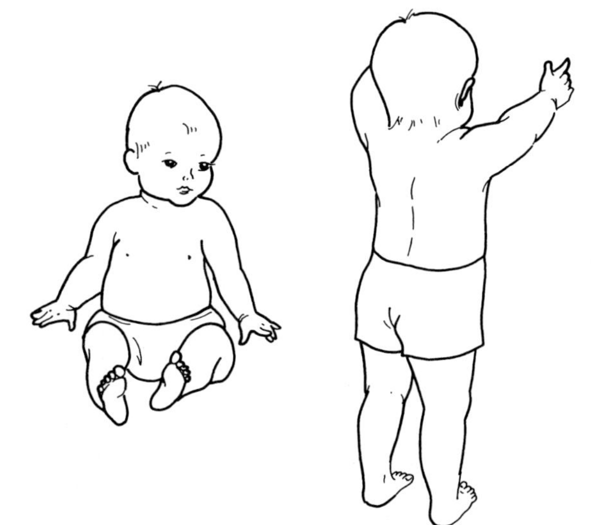

Fig. 4 Neuromotor patterns (2).

positions and movement patterns used by the infant as he advances towards controlled movement.

Fully developed controlled movement is dependent on a fully functioning brain. However, the newborn brain is not fully developed, and must be programmed if it is to direct normal movement. This is what happens in the early months after birth.

DEVELOPMENT OF THE POSTURAL REFLEX MECHANISM

If the development of the postural reflex mechanism, described above in the normal infant, is not understood it is impossible to make a reasoned and realistic approach to stroke rehabilitation.

As mentioned in Chapter 1, the postural reflex mechanism consists of three main factors: normal postural tone and its adjustment, normal reciprocal innervation and normal patterns of coordination. This is the mechanism which we do not have at birth. It develops in the infant stages of kicking, rolling, crawling, kneeling and standing, or along the parallel lines of rolling to sitting to standing, and rolling to prone lying to propping to crawling to standing.

LEVELS OF REFLEX ACTIVITY

As the development of the postural reflex mechanism becomes familiar we can recognize the different levels of reflex activity:

1. spinal
2. tonic
3. basal
4. cortical.

The postural reflex mechanism develops from tonic reflex levels and labyrinthine reflexes. The spinal and tonic levels lead to the basal level, where righting reflexes and equilibrium responses are developed. The latter two mechanisms include a cortical element and, as soon as they are thoroughly established, the cortical level (with voluntary responses and learned skills) takes over. Note that all levels from spinal upwards can be modified, but basal response is necessary before cortical response can be effective. This important point must be understood and used as a guideline when working out the rehabilitation programme for individual patients, relating the exercise programme to the level of recovery.

Tonic reflexes

Tonic reflexes produce involuntary changes in muscle tone in response to stimulation of sensory nerve endings, the exteroceptors and proprioceptors. Of these we are most concerned with stimulation of the proprioceptors in response to changes of the body's position in space (e.g. by rolling), with associated changes in pressure on soft tissues and weight transference.

There are three distinct types of tonic reflex:

1. The positive supporting response which gives an increase in extensor tone in a limb bearing weight.
2. The negative supporting response which gives a decrease in extensor tone when weight is taken off a limb.
3. The withdrawal response which gives an increase in flexor tone in response to undesirable stimulation.

These are involuntary reflex happenings but must be understood if a realistic approach to re-education of the postural reflex mechanism is to be undertaken.

Tonic labyrinthine and tonic neck reflexes

These are stereotyped primitive responses which are modified or overruled at higher levels when the postural reflex mechanism is fully established. They play a very important role in stroke rehabilitation.

The tonic labyrinthine reflex obviously depends on an intact spinal cord and brain stem. The receptor organs are the labyrinthine canals of the inner ear. As the afferent pathway influences the vestibular nuclei, causing these neurones to send excitatory impulses to fusimotor fibres of the extensor muscles, and so increasing the reaction to stretch stimuli, this reflex increases extensor tone. Because of this reflex, the position of the head has a fundamental bearing on muscle tone.

The tonic neck reflexes relate to the position of the cervical spine and, again, the afferent pathways influence the vestibular nuclei, but the pattern of increased muscle tone differs according to the alteration in the position of the cervical spine. Two quite distinct patterns may be demonstrated.

1. The symmetrical tonic neck reflex results from flexion or extension of the cervical spine. With flexion, extensor tone increases in the lower limbs and decreases in the upper limbs. With extension, extensor tone decreases in the lower limbs and increases in the upper limbs.
2. The asymmetrical tonic neck reflex is related to rotation of the cervical spine. For example, if the head is turned to the left there is an increase in extensor tone in the limbs of the left side and a decrease in extensor tone in the limbs of the right side, and vice versa if the head is turned to the right.

Basal: righting reflexes and equilibrium responses

A righting response is a combination of righting reflexes, while equilibrium responses are very complex mechanisms which develop from righting responses. In a book of this length, only a simple description is possible.

The head righting reaction follows movement of the head in space with correction of eye level in response to disturbance of the labyrinth. The head rights, movement of the cervical spine stretches the neck muscles and triggers off the reflex mechanism which aligns the head, neck and trunk. This leads to controlled rolling, controlled rolling to sitting, and finally to the ability to rotate within the body's axis and, therefore, to controlled movement, rotation being a necessary component of normal movement.

Equilibrium responses follow in the development pattern. Tonic reflexes, which cause changes in muscle tone with weight transference, combine with righting responses to give automatic shifts in tone all over the body, which relate to position changes, making possible the patterns of movement necessary for daily living. These are the responses which are required to carry out any action smoothly against gravity, to 'place' a limb and to 'hold' at rest, to 'hold' against gravity and to maintain balance. Equilibrium responses, therefore, include shifts in muscle tone with compensating movements to allow the body to meet any altering situation caused by changes of position or environment. When fully developed, equilibrium responses allow us to support our weight over a fixed base, or, if necessary, to find a new base. They allow us to 'prop' over a fixed base; to maintain this fixed base while reaching out in any direction; to maintain balance against an external opposing force, and to regain lost balance by reaching out, hopping or sidestepping.

Cortical: voluntary responses and learned skills

It is important to note that all reflex levels from spinal to cortical can be modified but, to emphasize once more, righting reflexes and equilibrium responses must be established before cortical level can be effective. Attempting to take a short cut in stroke rehabilitation, and neglecting to establish righting reflexes and equilibrium responses, will leave a missing link in the recovery chain and ruin the patient's chances of returning to a normal life.

FOLLOWING NEURODEVELOPMENTAL PATTERNS FOR REHABILITATION

The antigravity mechanism of the human body, and in particular the reflexes mentioned above, which are so closely concerned with obtaining an upright position and correct body alignment, must be used in stroke rehabilitation if it is to be effective. Wherever there is a regression of motor skills to a more primitive level with loss of controlled movement, loss of equilibrium responses, possible perceptual difficulty and loss of sensory discrimination, it is necessary to go back to the beginning and start rebuilding on a firm foundation.

It makes sound sense to think of the reflex arc as the basic functional unit of the nervous system and to seriously consider a course of rehabilitation which builds on this basic unit. However, to follow this line of thought, and to transfer the theory of rehabilitating the brain damage of stroke by following neurodevelopmental patterns, will not lead to any significant improvement if the barriers to normal development are not addressed. Of these barriers the greatest are developing spasticity and sensory loss. Normal movement depends on close interaction between sensory and motor events. One may, by all means, use motor development patterns but only if, at the same time, a way is found to break down these barriers to normal development.

THE PROBLEM OF DEVELOPING SPASTICITY

In all effective rehabilitation of the stroke patient it is essential to re-establish the normal postural reflex mechanism, which includes cortical control, but this cannot be done unless developing spasticity is contained while rehabilitation is undertaken. In other words, with the stroke patient, cortical control is lost; the static postural reflexes are no longer under cortical control and are no longer integrated into functional movement patterns. The result is abnormal tonic reflex activity giving the typical picture of the spastic hemiplegia.

In any assessment of motor disability following a stroke, where the assessor has a thorough knowledge of the working of the postural reflex mechanism, it is possible to establish the level of disability at which to begin the rehabilitation programme. In order to achieve full motor recovery it is frequently found to be indeed necessary to start at spinal level.

The rehabilitation concept presented here is eclectic, gathered from many sources, put together over a period of forty years in the clinical field and judged and verified by the rehabilitation results obtained. It offers a clear way ahead for the stroke victim in a step-by-step guide, and begins by facing up to the problem of developing spasticity.

A hands-on examination of many patients immediately after the onset of a stroke strongly suggests that there is no spasticity but, from day 1 of onset of the stroke, it begins to develop until, in many cases, it becomes the insurmountable barrier to restoration of normal movement. Could this development be prevented? If it has already started could its continuance be prevented? Or, if it has been allowed to develop until fixed spasticity patterns have taken over, is there any way of tackling the severe rehabilitation problem this presents?

Prevention is better than cure but, to understand the problem and its possible solution, one must go back to basic neurology and find out why spasticity develops and why it follows fixed patterns.

Considering the normal should suggest ways of dealing with the abnormal. In this instance, it leads to suggested measures which make it possible to plan a physical rehabilitation programme that provides a reasonable chance of recovery of balanced muscle tone and normal movement. Such a programme should not be stereotyped; it is difficult to find two patients who present in exactly the same way. The physiotherapist should carefully assess each patient and a rehabilitation programme must be based on the findings. However, if there is to be a reasonable hope of establishing an ongoing recovery programme the basic neurological facts must be taken into account. Effective measures must be taken to overcome abnormal muscle tone.

Normal muscle tone is balanced. In the brain damage of stroke, muscle tone is no longer balanced. The reciprocal innervation between agonists and antagonists necessary for normal movement has been disrupted. Is it possible to restore the balance produced by reciprocal innervation?

Normal muscle tone is based on the reflex arc. The stretch reflex is the key to the problem. In the example given in Chapter 1, to extend the elbow the stronger antagonist (biceps) must relax to allow the movement to take place. Initially biceps also contracts to resist the opposing contraction of triceps. In normal muscle tone the stretch reflex relayed to the biceps is inhibited to allow normal movement to take place (see Fig. 1). It is this inhibitory input from the brain which is missing after a stroke. (Note that I did not have positive confirmation of this, backed by scientific research, in my early practice in the clinical field. It was simply a hypothesis to be taken on trust, and resulting from a reasoned approach to the rehabilitation problems, which led to a logical conclusion.)

Normal muscle tone is more marked in the antigravity muscles. Where normal muscle tone has been more marked in the antigravity muscles before a stroke, it is logical to suppose that excessive antigravity muscle tone will present a very difficult rehabilitation problem after a stroke. This problem must be faced and an effective method of dealing with it must be found. The missing inhibitory input from cortical level must now be offered by some outside influence which can effectively control and correct the patient's imbalance of muscle tone while rehabilitation is undertaken. This does not apply only to movement of one joint (as in the elbow; consideration must be given to the whole body and to complete patterns of movement throughout the whole body.

AN EFFECTIVE REHABILITATION PROGRAMME

Those who set out on the difficult task of presenting a hopeful and effective rehabilitation programme are faced with the problem of restoring movement patterns other than those produced by reflexes which are no longer under cortical control. Can therapists really offer an effective way of dealing with this enormous problem?

It seemed to me that it had to be possible to establish resting and exercise regimens which would follow developmental patterns and, at the same time, inhibit and control the dominating antigravity muscles by avoiding extension patterns at all times (except for the forearm and hand). Furthermore, I was not prepared to abandon the neurodevelopmental exercise patterns taught to me in the clinical field by Professor Norman Dott (Hendrie & Macleod 1991).

If the stroke patient is to follow the neurodevelopmental patterns, developing spasticity must be held at a minimum, or the dominant tone must be inhibited as the nondominant (or low) tone is increased while rehabilitation goes forward. A way must be found to influence and control the distribution of muscle tone while treatment is undertaken, and successful treatment must be based on a continuing reliable assessment of the individual patient's state of muscle tone.

Summing up. The pattern of spasticity in the stroke patient bears a direct relationship to the dominating reflexes, and these are the reflexes which are modified at cortical level when the postural reflex mechanism is fully established. Muscle tone is always stronger in the antigravity muscles and after brain damage from stroke the developing patterns of spasticity bear a direct relationship to these muscles.

GUIDELINES FOR PLANNING REHABILITATION

The rehabilitation programme aims at restoring the postural reflex mechanism and, therefore, at restoring postural tone, leading to normal reciprocal innervation and normal patterns of movement.

It is helpful to have guidelines on which to base a positive and dynamic progress plan. For example:

1. Make a sound and positive decision about which muscles must be considered as the main antigravity supports.
2. Decide where and how to make a start.
3. Look at total tonal patterns and consider associated reactions.
4. Consider ways and means of introducing inhibitory practice.
5. What can the programme offer where there is marked proprioceptive loss?

Considered in this way, there is a logical and practical course to be followed.

1. MAKE A SOUND AND POSITIVE DECISION ABOUT WHICH ARE THE MAIN ANTIGRAVITY MUSCLES

The chief muscles by which the erect posture is maintained will be closely involved in extension, which will include trunk to shoulder and trunk to hip. For these gross movement patterns there are two main muscles to consider: latissimus dorsi and gluteus maximus.

Latissimus dorsi is a large triangular-shaped muscle which has its origin in the posterior part of the iliac crest and the spinous processes of the lumbar and lower thoracic vertebrae. It passes obliquely upwards across the back and under the arm to be inserted by a narrow tendon into the floor of the bicipital groove of the humerus (hence the shoulder involvement). It is the broadest muscle of the back. With its extensive origins it covers a large area of the trunk and assists in extension of the trunk and shoulder. Its action on the shoulder is very important. It extends, retracts and *inwardly rotates* the shoulder, drawing the arm downwards and backwards.

Gluteus maximus forms the main bulk of the buttock. It originates from the outer surface of the iliac bone and the sacrum, and is inserted into the upper end of the femur. It is the muscle chiefly concerned with the maintenance of erect posture and this explains why it is much more developed in man than in animals. It extends, retracts and *outwardly rotates* the hip.

These are the two most powerful antigravity muscles in the human body. Clinical observation over a number of years strongly supports subjective evidence for the selection of these two major muscles as the main determinants of spasticity patterns. This is based on my clinical study, over a period of 8 years, offering late treatment to severely affected stroke patients. Shoulder and hip disability included fixed inward rotation of the shoulder and fixed outward rotation of the hip in a large majority of cases examined. Also, because of the size and origins of these two antigravity muscles, lateral shortening of the trunk on the affected side was also found when late treatment was offered.

It is not surprising that these large muscles which together cover such a large area of the posterior aspect of the trunk dominate extensor patterns. Is that all that has to be said, or need we go further in an attempt to establish extensor patterns, or should other muscles be included? Practical clinical experience must help to establish the necessary answers.

2. DECIDE WHERE AND HOW TO MAKE A START

Examination of spasticity patterns found in the trunk several months after the onset of a stroke frequently reveals an immobile scapula, with trunk shortening and side flexion to the affected side, plus extension, retraction and inward rotation of the shoulder. In the lower trunk there is a similar problem with hip extension, retraction and, in this case, outward rotation. In other words these spasticity patterns are set by the uninhibited actions of latissimus dorsi and gluteus maximus because the necessary antigravity inhibitory input from the brain is missing. Reciprocal innervation is out of control.

Starting with the trunk and deciding how to take action to avoid developing spasticity, careful inhibiting positioning (see below) must be included in the rehabilitation programme to prevent excessive development of the antigravity tone which would lead to lateral shortening of the trunk and severe shoulder problems. The corrective positions used are those which oppose the action of latissimus dorsi. Likewise, developing spasticity of the hip must be inhibited by positioning in patterns which oppose the action of gluteus maximus.

Stroke disability is all too often thought of as loss of normal movement in the affected arm and leg. However, with the large trunk origins of the chief muscles which maintain man's erect posture, we cannot afford to neglect the disability which occurs in the trunk.

3. LOOK AT TOTAL TONAL PATTERNS AND CONSIDER ASSOCIATED REACTIONS

As long as it is possible to find in any 'caring' situation a stroke patient who has been instructed to struggle to perform a task with a disabled hand, while the rest of the arm is held fast in ever-increasing spasticity, we must recognize that there is still a great need for further education concerning the brain damage which has to be faced as a result of cerebrovascular accidents. Such practices cannot result in normal function of the hand; indeed, in such a case, because of associated reactions the patient is being encouraged to increase his disability.

There is a great and urgent need for better understanding in the following two areas:

a. The neurological result where the inhibitory input from the brain no longer has any influence on the maintenance of normal muscle tone.

b. Of equal importance, there is a great need for full understanding of total tonal patterns. This understanding must include normal patterns, as well as the abnormal patterns resulting from the lack of inhibitory control and, therefore, the lack of reciprocal innervation.

4. CONSIDER WAYS AND MEANS OF INTRODUCING INHIBITORY PRACTICE

First, return to the shoulder joint, remembering that the extensive and very strong antigravity muscle, latissimus dorsi, is now in a state where the stretch reflex is no longer inhibited and, with release from cortical control, spasticity will develop and will follow the dominant pattern set by latissimus dorsi.

Next consider the hip, and here the strongest antigravity muscle in the whole of the body is to be found. The main action of gluteus maximus is to thrust the body into the strong extension pattern used to move from sitting to standing. It therefore has a dominant effect on the hip joint.

These two major muscles must be inhibited after a stroke, and some ways of doing this are considered in the final section of this chapter and in some of the following chapters.

5. WHAT CAN THE PROGRAMME OFFER WHERE THERE IS MARKED PROPRIOCEPTIVE LOSS?

As the programme develops, sensory input increases having, for example, a positive effect on muscle proprioceptors by altering weight distribution as rolling routines are practised. However, where marked proprioceptive loss is present, there is a vital need to introduce other treatment techniques. Chapter 4, on the use of pressure techniques, and Chapter 5, on sensory loss and the importance of assessment, present treatment methods which have a positive effect on recovery of the missing function this deficit presents.

ADDRESSING THE PROBLEM OF SPASTICITY

THE TYPICAL SPASTICITY PATTERN

As might be expected, a typical spasticity pattern (Fig. 5) includes the following:

1. Retraction of the affected shoulder with depression and inward rotation.
2. Forearm flexion, usually accompanied by pronation.

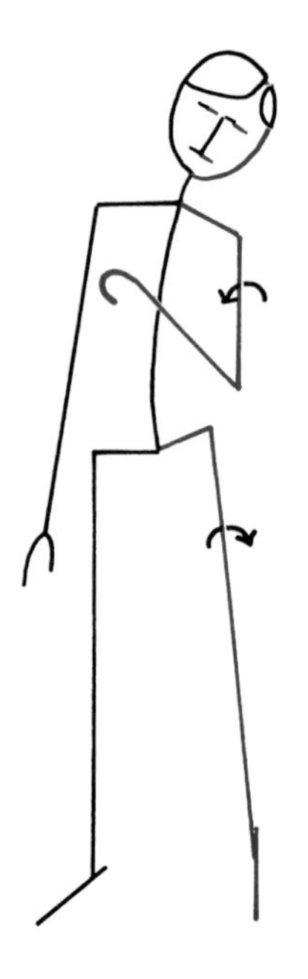

Fig. 5 The spasticity pattern.

3. Finger flexion with adduction.
4. Retraction of the pelvis with outward rotation of the leg.
5. Hip, knee and ankle extension with inversion and plantar flexion of the ankle.
6. Lateral flexion to the affected side.

This pattern may be expected to develop after the onset of a stroke. In the typical stroke patient, spasticity follows the usual brief initial flaccid stage, but develops all too quickly unless something can be done to prevent it. This is the situation that challenges all of us who set out to rehabilitate stroke patients. It should be possible to re-educate missing function in many cases, by early, intensive and repetitive treatment involving rolling, prone lying, elbow propping, kneeling, crawling and so on, working up through the levels of reflex activity. However, while this programme is carried out, it is a sad fact that developing spasticity usually outstrips rehabilitation and effectively puts an end to all worthwhile treatment. Also, antigravity for the forearm and hand is a flexion pattern while for the rest of the body it is an extension pattern; this is the single most important cause of our very poor record in recovery of arm function after a stroke. It is not easy to inhibit the forearm flexion pattern while flexion is encouraged in the rest of the body.

POSITIONING AND THE ANTISPASTICITY PATTERN

Developing spasticity must be held at a minimum while rehabilitation is carried out. However, as long as there is lack of cortical control, spasticity will develop.

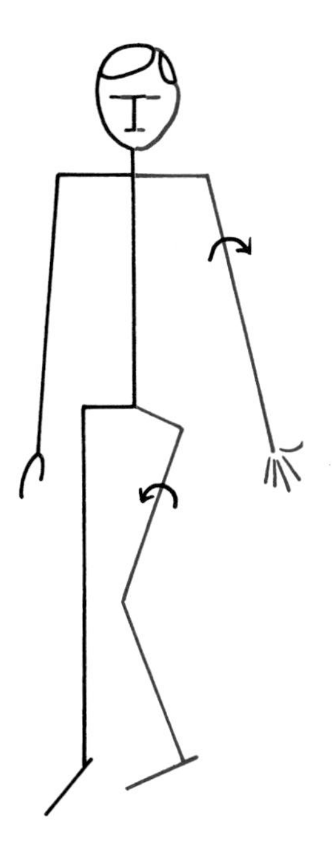

Fig. 6 The antispasticity pattern.

This seems to be a vicious circle, but there is a way out. The answer is to be found in 'positioning', that is, using the antispasticity (or recovery) pattern at all times. From the day of onset the patient must be placed in the anti-spasticity pattern, and all exercise must lead into recovery patterns.

If the typical spasticity pattern (Fig. 5) has been recognized, understanding the antispasticity or recovery pattern ought not to present any difficulty. It is quite simply the pattern which is in direct opposition to the spasticity pattern and is shown in Figure 6. Again, as might be expected, the positions of the shoulder and hip are of supreme importance, to counteract the strong action of latissimus dorsi and gluteus maximus.

The antispasticity pattern consists of the following:

1. Protraction of the shoulder with outward rotation. (*Note*: the thumb should always point outward away from the body.)
2. Forearm extension with supination.
3. Finger extension with abduction of the thumb.
4. Protraction of the hip with inward rotation.
5. Hip, knee and ankle flexion.
6. Elongation of the trunk on the affected side.

THE IMPORTANCE OF CORRECTIVE POSITIONING

So, it will be seen that the antigravity spasticity pattern in the stroke patient, as in all neurological conditions, involves total patterns of movement and, therefore, if allowed to develop, will prevent re-education of all normal patterns of voluntary movement on the affected side. The reflex activity of muscles which act as antagonists against gravity is no longer controlled, and the resulting hyperactivity gives the typical spasticity pattern as described above. In the stroke patient we talk about the *synergic pattern of tonic contraction* which results from hypertonic, or excessive, muscle tone in the antigravity muscles, giving the typical spasticity pattern which also lacks rotation. In other words, the fine balance between reciprocal relaxation and co-contraction is thrown out of gear, and the synergists, which normally contract and relax in conjunction with the prime movers crossing more than one joint, upset normal coordination because the stretch reflex lacks the vital inhibitory input from the brain.

It is this developing spasticity with loss of rotation that must be held in check by diligent positioning, using inhibitory patterns at all times. Is this possible? Not unless those who care for the stroke patient understand the importance of corrective positioning, which should be part of the recovery programme and should be started as early as day 1 of onset of the stroke. Even the unconscious patient will be turned from side to side every 2 hours and this must be done correctly. If not, and the patient survives, it will be found later that already symptoms of the agony shoulder have begun.

POSITIONING

Positioning is used to influence the distribution of muscle tone. Therefore, positioning must be used correctly at all times during exercise sessions and during resting periods; this means 24 hours a day. This will only be possible if those who care for the patient understand the rehabilitation needs of each patient. Note that this specialized care, once it is understood, is not complicated or difficult to undertake. It makes full recovery possible in many cases and also makes for easy handling with the least stress for the patient and for the nurse.

Understanding the distribution of muscle tone and relating this to the patient's needs leads to a reasoned and corrective approach to stroke care.

THE RESTING POSITIONS

One must begin by establishing total patterns when the body is at rest.

1. Lying on the back (supine) increases extensor tone.
2. Lying on the front (prone) increases flexor tone.
3. Lying on the side is the most neutral position.
4. Movement of the sound side increases tone in the affected side.

How can these four points be used to best advantage to assist in recovery of normal muscle tone?

1. Lying on the back (supine) increases extensor tone. Wherever possible patients should not be left lying flat on their backs. The total inhibiting position used to prevent the build-up of unwanted antigravity tone is a flexion

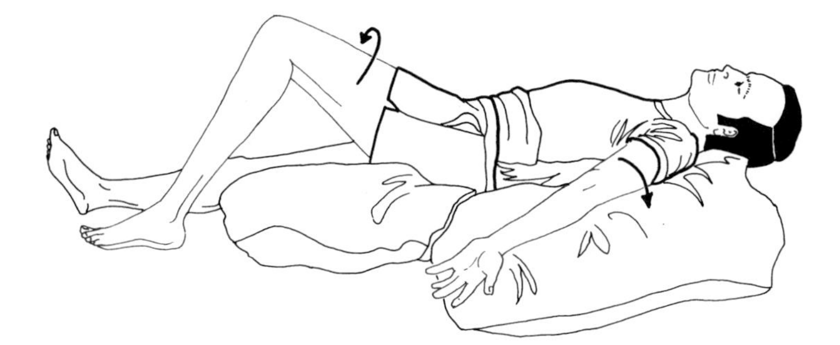

Fig. 7 Lying on the back.

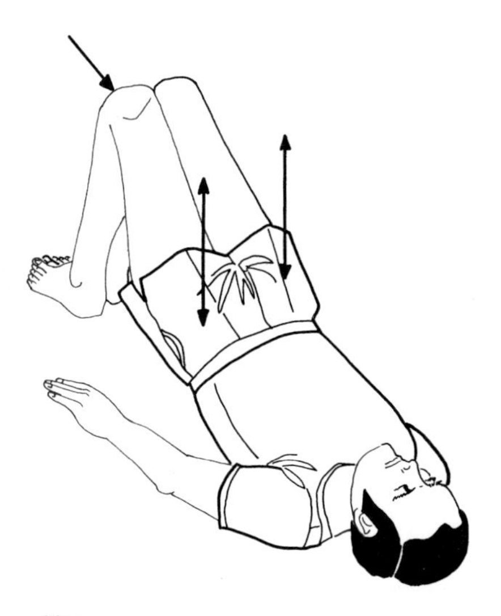

Fig. 8 The bridging position.

pattern, except for the forearm and hand where the opposite is true, and here extension is the inhibiting pattern. So, lying on the back can be therapeutic for forearm and hand but not for the rest of the body. If or when this position has to be used the patient should be supported by pillows during resting (Fig. 7) or, once the position is established, it may be used in exercise sessions without pillow support and with both knees flexed (Fig. 8).

2. *Lying on the front* (prone) increases flexor tone. This position is not used in the early days after a stroke. A beneficial way of using the prone position in exercise routines, at a later stage of the recovery programme, is suggested in Chapter 4.

3. *Lying on the side* is the most neutral position.

Lying on the *sound* side (Fig. 9) well supported by pillows is the most neutral and the most comfortable position for the stroke patient. The supporting pillows must maintain the inhibiting arm pattern but, as rolling onto the side is a total flexion pattern, the affected leg falls easily into the required flexion

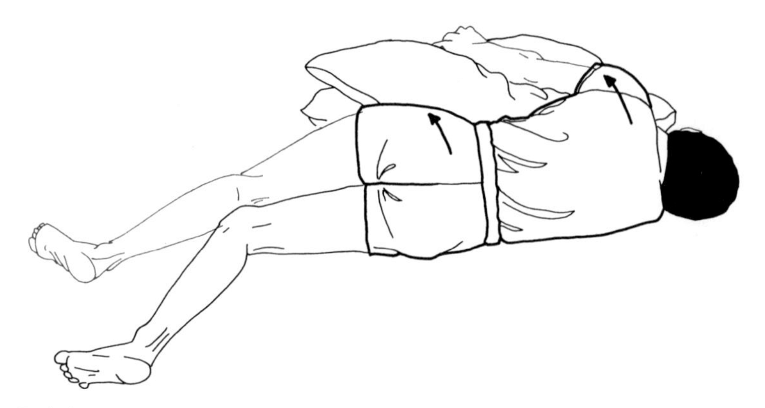

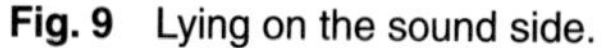

Fig. 9 Lying on the sound side.

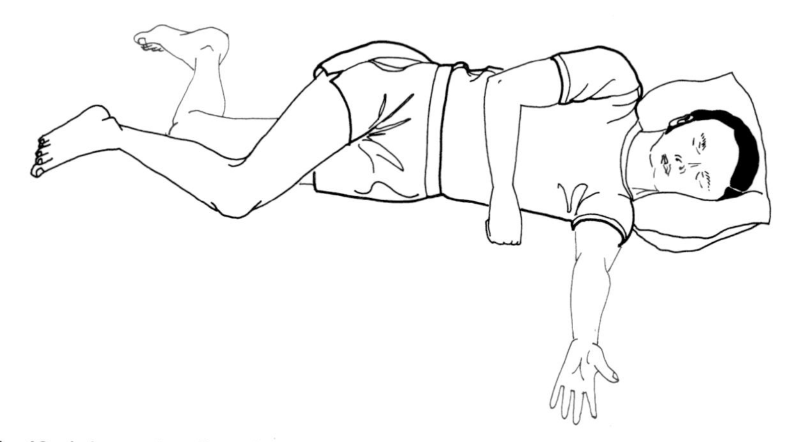

Fig. 10 Lying on the affected side.

pattern. Long clinical practice has shown this to be the preferred position for sleep at night.

Lying on the *affected* side (Fig. 10) is also useful, particularly where there is a need for more sensory input, but adequate care must be taken of the affected shoulder which must be placed well forward in protraction with the elbow, wrist and fingers extended. If in doubt about any of these important positions study Figures 7, 9 and 10.

Note: At no time should the stroke patient be rolled over onto a trapped shoulder (this is one of the common ways of starting off the agony shoulder syndrome). To avoid this the shoulder must be maintained in outward rotation with protraction (see Fig. 10).

4. Movement of the sound side increases tone in the affected side. Uninhibited associated reactions take over and tonal overflow in the affected side follows the unwanted spasticity pattern. Knowing this to be the case, how is it possible for therapists to resort to the use of a walking stick on the sound side, as still frequently happens? All such practice should surely have been discarded but, sadly, this is not so. Where this outdated practice is used, it puts an end to all expectations of restoring normal postural tone.

Ensuring correct positioning

Figures 7–10 illustrate the four basic and essential inhibiting positions which should be used at all times when the patient is lying down and which, in the very early days of treatment, should be maintained by adequate pillow support. Treatment will not succeed if nurses are not taught the need for this careful positioning and are not integrated into the team approach. In many ways the nurse or the family carer is the most important person concerned with the patient's recovery in the early days and can monitor the positioning programme.

STABILIZATION OF POSITIONS

It is important to note that as rehabilitation goes ahead, each advancing position must be stabilized. It is particularly important to stabilize side-lying as in Figure 9 and the leg positions as in Figure 8 (the bridging position).

1. It is important to teach the patient to balance (or stabilize) in a position before asking him to move into that position. If the patient is afraid that he cannot balance in a position, he will not be able to move into that position because his movement will be inhibited by fear, and his progress will be considerably retarded.
2. Progress in stroke rehabilitation is made by working through a sequence of exercise progressions which closely follow the patterns of motor development as seen in the infant. All progressions are made from a specific starting position and the patient must be thoroughly stabilized in the required starting position before he moves into each advancing series of exercises.
3. Stability is usually obtained by asking the patient to hold a position against gentle pressure offered by the therapist. The skill of the therapist lies in her ability to use her manual contacts, and the pressure she applies to her patient, in the correct way to gain the response she requires. She is working to achieve postural stability for her patient and begins by helping him to establish stability of the head, neck and trunk. Therefore, in the early days, positioning of the limbs in the inhibiting pattern is of supreme importance so that associated reactions produced by the above technique will not step up a flow of unwanted tone in the limbs. Indeed, with correct positioning, the weak tonal pattern will be reinforced and increased. This adds up to very good practice.
4. Stabilizing must include weightbearing through both sides of the body in sitting, kneeling and standing; it is essential to make sure that stabilizing is never practised in a position of compensation, using the sound side of the body and neglecting the affected side. Corrective inhibiting positioning is used at all times to influence the distribution of the patient's muscle tone (Johnstone 1987).
5. Rhythmical stabilization is practised by giving steady static contractions of the muscle groups round the trunk or round the joints, in this case, the

proximal joints; the shoulder and hip, are attended to first. The static contractions are achieved by applying steady manual pressure from therapist to patient, the therapist using such commands as 'Don't let me move you!'. The pressure should be applied very slowly and should gradually build up as the muscles respond. A steady static contraction of one group of muscles is immediately followed by a similar contraction of the opposite group of muscles. The therapist's manual pressure should always build up slowly and withdraw slowly, no movement being allowed to take place (Knott & Voss 1968).

REFERENCES

Hendrie W F, Macleod D A D 1991 The Bangour story: a history of Bangour Village and general hospitals. Aberdeen University Press, Aberdeen

Johnstone M 1987 Restoration of motor function in the stroke patient, 3rd edn. Churchill Livingstone, Edinburgh

Knott M, Voss D 1968 Proprioceptive neuromuscular facilitation, 2nd edn. Harper and Row, New York

3

THE BASIC CONCEPT

BUILDING AN ACTIVE REHABILITATION PROGRAMME

Considering the neurological facts so far presented, it will be found that there is a possible and logical way to begin building a rehabilitation programme which should have a reasonable chance of obtaining sound progress towards motor recovery.

The inhibitory resting positions, if introduced in the very early days after the onset of a stroke, are frequently found to be easy to establish, provided there is adequate pillow support: a minimum of five pillows is required, one packed firmly into the small of the back for side-lying. Next one must stabilize all four positions (see Figs 7–10) and, wherever possible, hand over to the patient the care of his own limbs. If all those who care for stroke patients use the same inhibitory positions it is often surprising how quickly this can be achieved.

FUNDAMENTAL RULES

There are four basic rules which must be observed from the outset of treatment.

1. Start early after onset of the stroke. (Even the unconscious patient must be maintained in corrective positioning of shoulder and hip.)

2. Maintain corrective positioning at all times.

3. Everyone who has any dealings with the patient must be instructed in the corrective inhibiting positioning which is essential to recovery of normal movement. The patient learns to live in the patterns of recovery which are based on the inhibiting patterns.

4. As has already been said, start with the trunk. It is not possible to rehabilitate limbs on an unstable trunk.

All care should be taken to inhibit the development of unwanted excessive antigravity muscle tone. Taking into account that the main antigravity extensors of the trunk also control movement from trunk to shoulder and trunk to hip, the inhibitory resting positions are translated into therapeutic movement patterns which follow neuromotor development patterns.

USING ROTATIONAL PATTERNS

The patient must not be allowed to roll onto a weak shoulder which is trapped below his body weight in the damaging position of inward rotation with retraction. This will start the agony shoulder syndrome. The reasoning behind the need to use rotational patterns is logical and easily understood.

Those who have studied the movement patterns used in proprioceptive neuromuscular facilitation (PNF) will be well versed in the need to perform total movement patterns and not to consider isolated movement in one joint (Knott & Voss 1968). The same need is found in stroke care; we set out to re-educate total movement patterns. For example, the movement of flexion of the shoulder joint with outward rotation is completed with extension of the elbow, wrist and fingers; flexion of the hip with inward rotation continues with flexion of the knee and ankle. These two patterns are also the inhibiting limb patterns that are used in this rehabilitation programme. Those who are familiar with PNF will also understand how the PNF patterns may be used to great advantage, provided no movement pattern is used which does not work into the correct inhibiting rotation.

FOLLOWING A DEVELOPMENTAL SEQUENCE

Fetal movements are reflex movements and are the predecessors of all purposeful, coordinated actions. At birth the first movements are still primitive: eye movements, head turning, kicking, finger grasp and so on. Neurological development takes place in the following weeks and months, building on the spinal reflex arc and bringing in tonic neck reflexes, labyrinthine reflexes and equilibrium responses; the postural reflex mechanism is established when reflexes are integrated into normal movement under cortical control and purposeful, voluntary responses are established with learned skills following. This is the sequence rehabilitation will attempt to follow.

A TEAM APPROACH

The physiotherapist must dig deep to uncover other problems that will be encountered if this recovery programme is to have any hope of success.

There is a need for a team approach. This treatment concept deals with muscles and recovery of normal movement, and no one carer can go it alone. Continuing with this line of thought, and having suggested that it is essential to find answers which face up to the two great barriers to the recovery of physical ability (inhibitory loss and sensory loss), it makes sense to consider the problem of developing spasticity and to make this problem the first treatment priority. Much can be done to prevent the all too often rapid onset of spasticity. However, to do this with any real hope of success, therapists and nurses must work together, both using the same movement and resting patterns. Failure to do this will result in failure to achieve successful treatment results.

When this team integration is not achieved, it is usually because nurses have not been taught the need for corrective positioning. Alternatively, an often-repeated excuse is that nurses are far too busy and haven't time to undertake this sort of care. This does not make sense, particularly in the early days of treatment. Positioning the unconscious patient has already been mentioned. Where nurses and physiotherapists work as one it is frequently found that patients establish therapeutic movement patterns very quickly and do not increase the demands made on the nurse. Rather, the work of the nurse is considerably eased and independent movement takes over.

And what of the rest of the team? I believe all should understand the need to maintain inhibitory patterns. There is a right way and a wrong way for occupational therapists to position their stroke patients, a right way and a wrong way for speech therapists to seat their patients, and a right side and a wrong side for social workers to approach the patient's bed or chair. Perhaps most important of all, wherever possible a family member should be integrated into this team approach. As for the physician, he or she leads the team in clinical matters, and the team should be aware of other problems such as diabetes, blood pressure, possible cause of each stroke, exercise tolerance level and any drugs being prescribed with their possible side-effects. If there is a case for surgical intervention this should also be understood.

This begins to look like a team approach, but one weak link in the team can destroy the hope of optimum recovery for each individual patient. For example, for a therapist to give a good session of treatment dealing with the reduction of arm spasticity, and then to find the patient sitting eating lunch with the affected hand crossed over to the sound side of his body with his elbow flexed and inward rotation of his shoulder reduces the therapist to a state of despair. All through the lunch session, because the hemiplegic arm is not in the inhibiting pattern, with every movement of the sound side associated reactions are increasing the spasticity tone.

Until this basic principle is understood, stroke rehabilitation (so called) will have a very poor outcome and is in danger of being judged as useless.

THE RATIONALE FOR STARTING WITH THE TRUNK

It should not be thought that the reason for starting with the trunk is a belief that control must be gained proximally before distally, and that this assumption is based on a strictly hierarchical view of motor control which some neurologists no longer support.

In the context of this book, proximal to distal recovery grew out of a need to re-establish the balanced muscle tone on which all normal movement depends. In normal movement, the preparatory postural adjustments, which take place to ensure that the destabilizing effect of the following voluntary movement is counterbalanced, must be dependent on normal muscle tone. Our aim is to rebuild a normal postural reflex mechanism. To do this, the control of antigravity muscle tone was seen as a top priority and, in clinical practice, this led to a firm conviction that the strongest antigravity muscles in man which concern our rehabilitation concept are those which thrust him upright into the standing position.

As a result, the need to start with the trunk was the obvious way forward, while the ongoing programme led to the natural progression of proximal to distal. I set out to monitor a rehabilitation programme which would control associated reactions and shift abnormal tonal patterns back to normal.

QUESTIONS AND ANSWERS CONCERNING MAT WORK

Why use mat work?

There are two main reasons.

1. Mat work provides the only possible way of following through the sequence of motor development as seen in the human infant.
2. Mat work is of particular value to the patient with limited stability because it provides:

- a wide base
- a low centre of gravity
- a sense of security.

Should the mat be on the floor?

The answer to this question is that it is usually a case of making do with whatever is available. Usually, where the question of cost has to be considered, the mat is placed on the floor. A large floor area that can accommodate a number of mats can be very useful, allowing several patients to be treated at the same time. There must be a ready source of pillows to be used where necessary to maintain the vital inhibiting patterns, which must be maintained at all times.

Are there any advantages in having a high mat?

Certainly, particularly in the early days of treatment. A high mat is more readily accessible, making patient handling much easier in the beginning, the area and height being suitable for sitting, for rolling and for training rolling to sitting. It is important to make sure the patient feels safe and not in danger of falling off the high mat on to the floor. The space from the high mat to the floor can seem like a yawning chasm to an early stroke patient.

A BROAD OUTLINE OF THE TREATMENT PLAN

NORMAL MOVEMENT

It is necessary to understand normal movement.

Normal movement depends on the following factors:

1. Normal tone: it must be neither too weak nor too strong.
2. Normal patterns of movement, as developed from the primitive reflex movement present at birth, to weightbearing with mobility and skills. The progression can be described as: automatic – voluntary – selective. The true recovery of normal movement must include automatic movement.
3. Normal postural reflex mechanism. This includes:
   a. righting reactions
      —head righting
      —rotating within the body axis
   b. equilibrium responses
      —moving the body against a fixed support
      —protective extension
   c. reciprocal innervation
      —interplay between antagonistic pairs of muscles.

THE INITIAL PURPOSE OF TREATMENT

To make a beginning by establishing inhibiting positioning (see Figs 7–10).

Next comes simple muscle work, using gross patterns of movement involved in trunk rotation. The patient is rehabilitated into bilateral rotation of the trunk, outward rotation of the shoulder with extension of the elbow, wrist and fingers and inward rotation of the hip with flexion of the knee and ankle. The aim is to restore postural control; first, bring in righting reactions, head righting and rotating within the body axis are introduced.

To maintain the inhibiting arm pattern, the hands are clasped with fingers interlaced, palms held together, elbows straight and arms held forward at, or above, shoulder level (see Fig. 12) and the legs are flexed (see Fig. 8). All trunk rolling patterns will include the head and neck; tonic labyrinthine and tonic neck reflexes must be taken into account. Rolling also stimulates proprioceptors.

IMPORTANT POINTS

The following points should be remembered:

1. Stability of the limbs must not be the first priority. Limbs cannot be stabilized on an unstable trunk.
2. Start with the trunk but, at the same time, use total body inhibiting positions and patterns.
3. Postural stability of the head, neck and trunk must come first.
4. Postural tone depends on joint compression. With the exception of the stimuli received via the eyes and vestibular apparatus, one of the most powerful stimuli to postural balance and stability is compression, which is normally experienced when the body bears weight.
5. Muscle tone is influenced by the position of the head and altering positions in the inner ears. Movement of the head stimulates nerve endings within membranous sacs in the semicircular canals. These are fine epithelial cells with minute hair-like projections which are the special end organs concerned with equilibratory vestibular reflexes. They influence, first, the position of the eyes in relation to movements of the head through the connections of the vestibular nerves and their nuclei; and secondly, muscle tone through the vestibulospinal tracts (Johnston et al 1958). The vestibular system is closely involved with postural control of muscle tone in relation to gravitational forces. The importance of the position of the head cannot be stressed too often. This emphasizes the need to include rolling patterns in this specialized rehabilitation programme.
6. Concerning tonal flow, the hope is that all resting positions and movement patterns will stimulate proprioceptors and, at the same time, abnormal muscle tone will be shifted back to normal because inhibitory patterns are maintained and used at all times.
7. Neurodevelopmental patterns will be used, or, to update this term, 'developmental reflexive rehabilitation' will be used (McGlown 1990).

POSITIONS AND EXERCISE PATTERNS

Figures 11–21 show some of the advancing exercise patterns and positions that are used in building a rehabilitation programme with a team approach and with trained nurses and/or carers.

Figure 11 illustrates the hand holds used in early shoulder care to maintain mobility of the shoulder joint in outward rotation. The shoulder will remain in outward rotation as long as the patient's thumb points away from his body. It is important to note that if early shoulder elevation gives pain (and particularly in weight-bearing situations) the vital outward rotation has not been maintained.

It is surprising how many therapists continue to make mistakes here. If in doubt about the position, stand up, outwardly rotate your own shoulder so that your thumb points away from your body, then, without allowing any alteration in shoulder rotation, raise your arm above your head and you will find your thumb continues to point away from your body. (See Ch. 5, concerning the hemiplegic shoulder.)

Figure 12 illustrates early self-care for the shoulder joint. With hands clasped, elbows straight, palms pressed together and arms held at or above shoulder level, the arrow shows the direction of movement. (Note that this is also the arm position used for rolling over and over across a large floor mat.) When he is lying supine, remember that the patient's legs must be stabilized in the bridging position (see Fig. 8); pillow support will be necessary in the early treatment days.

The pillow support should be removed when rolling begins. Then, to start the roll over, the patient is encouraged to turn his eyes and then his head in the direction of the roll, following with his shoulders, arms and trunk. Rotation of the lower trunk inhibits spasticity in the lower half of the body and his legs will follow his body. Resting time should be spent in side-lying with adequate shoulder care. Never allow the patient to lie on a disabled shoulder which is trapped below his body in inward rotation. To do this is to start the agony shoulder syndrome, but, this will not happen if the patient maintains the hands clasped position with his arms straight as illustrated in Figure 12.

Note: Rolling to the affected side is usually easier than rolling to the sound side. This is because rolling to the sound side is led by the affected side. Initial tuition in rolling is required until the patient can take over and add this to his list of self-care exercises.

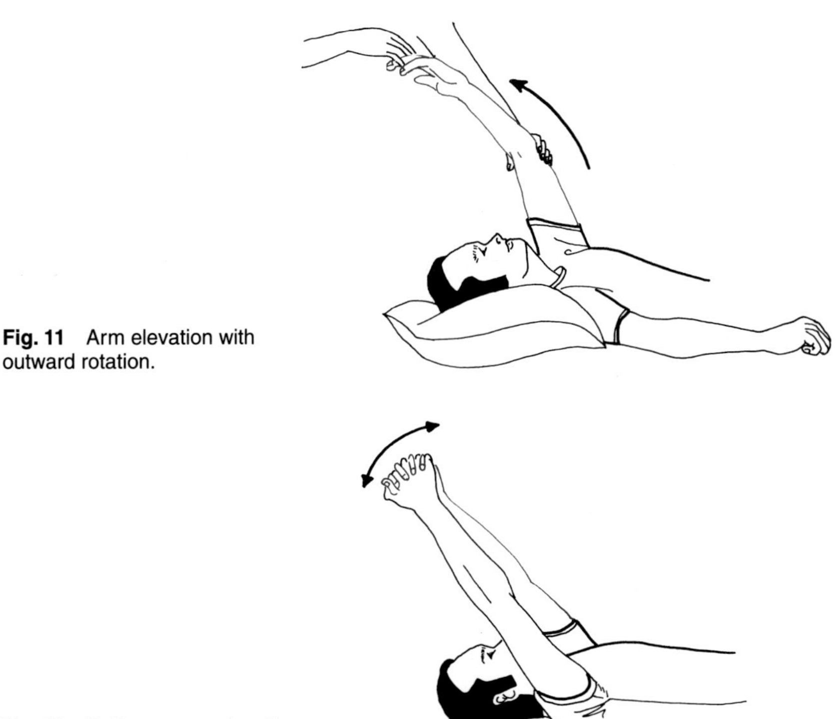

Fig. 11 Arm elevation with outward rotation.

Fig. 12 Self-care arm elevation.

Figure 13 illustrates hand holds used to maintain mobility of the scapula and the shoulder. The scapula should slide freely round the chest wall. Maintaining this free mobility will greatly assist the measures to be taken to promote shoulder recovery.

Note: At this stage of recovery, when lying supine in the bridging position (see Fig. 8), time should be spent on stabilizing the pelvis, and the affected leg must not be allowed to drift into outward rotation. Stabilize the pelvis by giving mild resistance through the iliac crests as the buttocks are lifted off the mat. Follow this with approximation down through the knees to the heels. Bridging is an essential exercise because it is used to maintain hip extension. The patient who remains unable to bridge will not later achieve a good walking gait.

Figure 14 illustrates rolling to sitting over the edge of the bed. The patient rolls towards his affected side to prop on his affected elbow, which is positioned by the helper so that weight is transmitted through a correctly positioned shoulder. The helper assists movement into the upright position as illustrated. It should be noted that the patient is not taught to hook his sound leg under his affected leg to assist the affected leg out of bed. This would spoil the whole sequence of the rolling patterns on which the rehabilitation programme is based.

To establish this movement sequence of rolling to sitting over the edge of the bed, two helpers are frequently needed: one behind the patient and one in front as he moves into sitting. However, with a team approach where all use the same method, balanced sitting on the bed is often established with surprising ease. Make sure that your patient feels safe in your hands at all times. He must never be put into a situation where he is afraid of falling.

Figure 15 suggests it is never too early to begin training in sitting balance. At this stage the patient is usually very unstable and here he is being asked to balance on the mattress, an unstable base. Balancing on an unstable base is introduced to the exercise programme at a later date; at the present stage the patient may feel very unsafe and the helper must give the support which will make him feel safe. As illustrated here she stands in front of him using her knees to support his knees and her hand holds to add to his feeling of safety and to begin to use gentle stabilizing pressures.

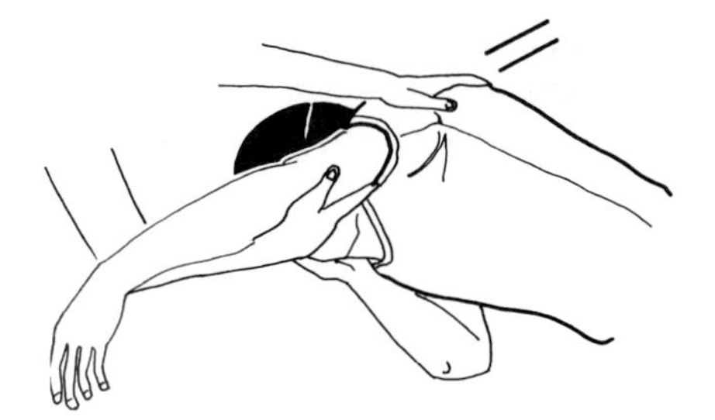

Fig. 13 Scapula movements.

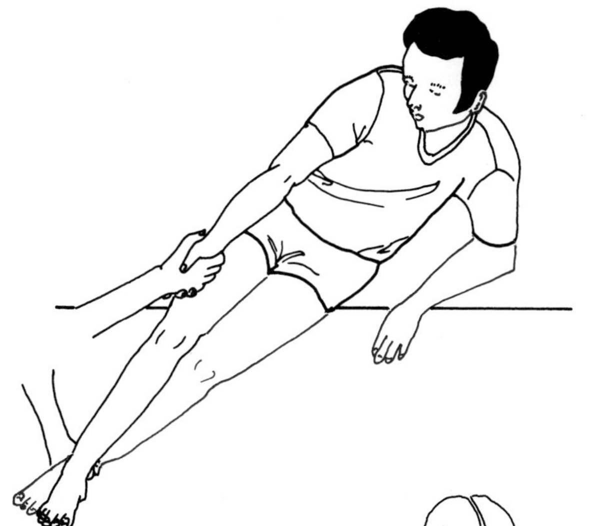

Fig. 14 Rolling to sitting.

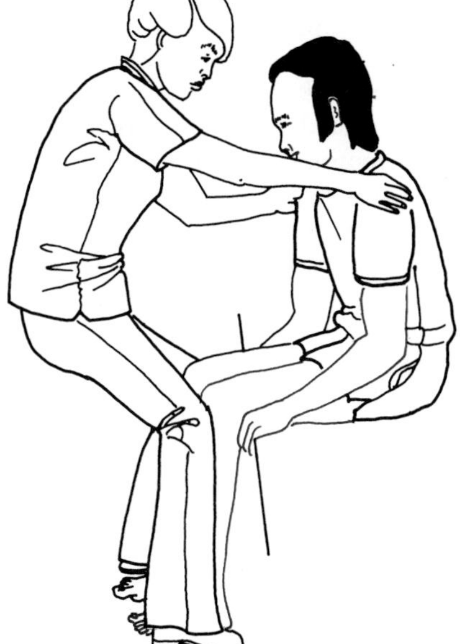

Fig. 15 Training in sitting balance.

Figure 16 shows maximum support for getting out of bed. Depending on the patient's medical state and guided by the physician, sitting on a chair, out of bed, will begin as soon as possible. The patient will quickly feel confident in transferring from bed to chair, carefully handled by the helper, with body contacts giving firm support. His trust and ability will increase quite quickly in many cases, provided every member of the team uses the same method of handling. Constant repetition of established movement patterns leads to increasing independence.

Figure 17 shows the furniture used to maintain inhibiting patterns when sitting out of bed. The red stripe down the middle of the table is used to remind the patient that he must not allow his affected hand to stray across the table towards his sound side, turning his affected shoulder into inward rotation. He must lean his weight through his forearm to a correctly positioned shoulder. His elbow must be on the table. Note that a cantilever table is very suitable because it does not interfere with the correct positioning of his feet.

Figure 18 demonstrates an early technique which can be used to train sitting to standing. As shown here the stool is much too low for early training. Start this training with a reasonably high chair with forearm support (see Fig. 17). The therapist supports and holds both of the patient's knees between her knees, supports his affected arm, holding it firmly in position with her own forearm and body, and encourages him to lean forward over her shoulder. Alternatively she may support his affected arm by placing it across her shoulder and asking him to hold it there with his other arm. Continuing to encourage him to lean forward she teaches him to stand up and sit down slowly. The patient should wear a suitable shoe with a non-slip sole. For her own self-care the therapist or nurse should at all times perform all lifts using the approved method which maintains a straight lumbar spine.

Note: In these early handling routines, if a patient is very severely disabled it may take two helpers to manage the early care, but if this is necessary, every effort should be made to maintain the inhibiting patterns and to follow the same routines. Always take particular care of the shoulder and hip positions.

At this stage, wherever possible, the patient should be taught to take care of his own limbs and to maintain the corrective inhibiting positioning. Self-care exercises are started. For example, while sitting he may be taught to clasp his hands, fingers interlaced, palms touching and to reach forwards and downwards to reach for the floor. As the advancing exercise programme progresses he will begin to take an active part in his own rehabilitation and to do more and more for himself.

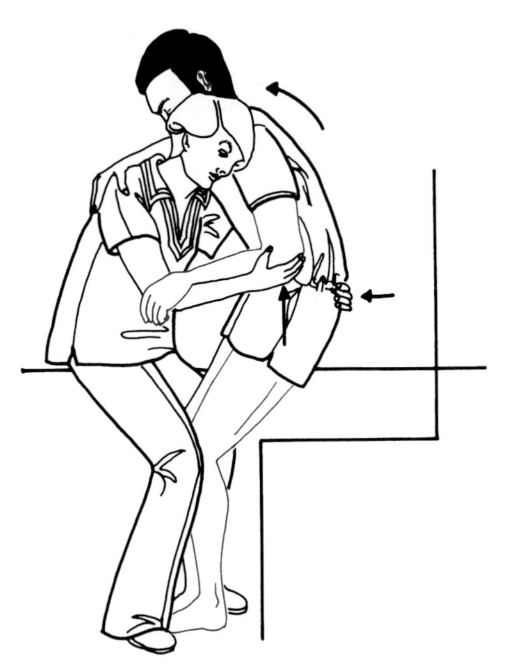

Fig. 16 Early transfer from bed to chair.

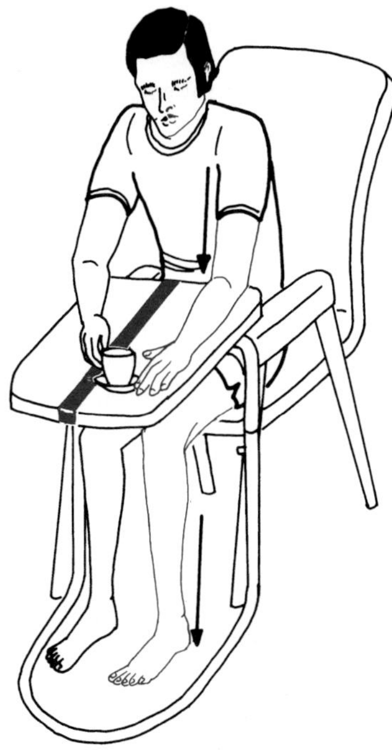

Fig. 17 Use inhibiting patterns at all times.

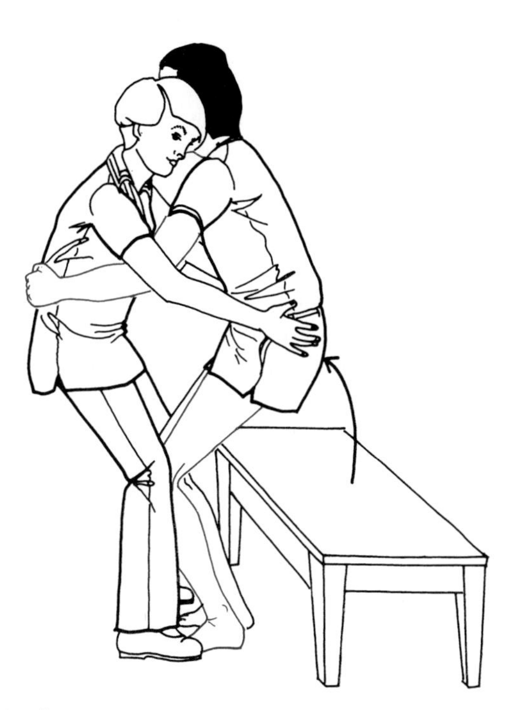

Fig. 18 Sitting to standing.

Figure 19 shows how to stabilize in sitting. It is useful to continue to use this technique after sitting balance has been established. Making use of PNF techniques, resistance is used to aid muscle contraction and motor control, to increase strength which adds to irradiation and reinforcement, with the response increasing as the stimuli increases (Adler et al 1993).

It will therefore be seen how vital it is to make sure that any of these techniques must only be practised while the patient is carefully positioned in inhibiting patterns. The pressure techniques the therapist uses will make a demand on her patient's affected side and, where careful inhibiting positioning is maintained, irradiation in the affected side will be diverted into low tonal patterns which directly oppose antigravity patterns.

It is also worth noting that a full understanding of PNF principles and movement patterns can be very useful, provided the therapist has enough knowledge to be able to discriminate between good and bad practice in stroke care. At no time must the limbs be used in diagonal patterns which move into contraindicated rotations.

In the text of this book 'overflow of tone' equates to 'irradiation'. We are dealing with muscle tone and an attempt to shift it from abnormal back to normal. Much of the success of this treatment concept depends on the therapist's ability to divert tonal overflow into inhibiting patterns. 'Approximation' is the compression of the trunk on an extremity. This technique is used extensively in the motor recovery programme and should be considered under any of three headings: 'approximation', 'compression' or 'weightbearing'.

Figure 19 demonstrates three distinct ways of gaining a required response.

1 & 2. This technique increases the low tonal pattern in the arm and directly stimulates joint proprioceptors in the elbow. Again this demonstrates the need to work through inhibiting patterns and here the therapist increases the stimuli by adding to the pressure down through the shoulder to the hand.

3. Gentle pressure to the back of the head stimulates tonic neck extension. The tonic neck reflexes relate to the position of the cervical spine. With cervical extension, extensor tone decreases in the lower limbs and increases in the upper limbs. In this instance the increased tone in the upper limbs, as a direct response to the demand placed at the back of the head, stimulates an extensor thrust through the arms. To increase the response, increase the stimuli. This is done by applying pressure to the back of the head, which will also direct cervical extension on into neck rotation towards the affected side.

It becomes increasingly clear that teaching on stroke rehabilitation should include study of the levels of reflex activity.

4. The technique shown here illustrates the maxim: 'Place your demand where you want your response', another PNF principle. In this instance the need is to transfer weight laterally over to the affected side and down through the affected arm. As shown, the therapist places her hand on the lateral aspect of the affected shoulder to give lateral pressure, and the patient responds by resisting this pressure and transferring his weight over to his affected side until balanced sitting is established. It is bad practice to attempt to achieve and maintain an upright trunk by putting pressure on his sound side and pulling him upright. His response to this is to resist the pressure and fall further over

to his sound side. The skill of the therapist lies in her ability to use hand holds and pressures correctly, to gain the required response. The hemiplegic patient is approached and handled from his affected side.

Cross-facilitation is used. To cross-facilitate is to work with the sound side of the body across the midline to the affected side, to initiate bilateral activity. Working in the clinical field with a hands-on approach, tonal patterns can be felt by the therapist. Rolling over to the affected side gives an increase in tonal flow (irradiation) into the hemiplegic side. The resulting increase in muscle activity occurs in the antigravity muscles, here the flexors of the elbow, wrist and fingers, and this indicates the urgent need to inhibit tonal overflow in the forearm and hand while, at the same time, encouraging a build-up of flexor tone in the rest of the body.

In the jargon of the physiotherapist, the stability of sustained posture is necessary for purposeful movement. In the recovery of the hemiplegic arm, this must mean stability of sustained posture of the arm held upward in space with the shoulder in outward rotation and elbow, wrist and fingers in extension. If this is to be obtained, the need is to step up tone in this forearm extension

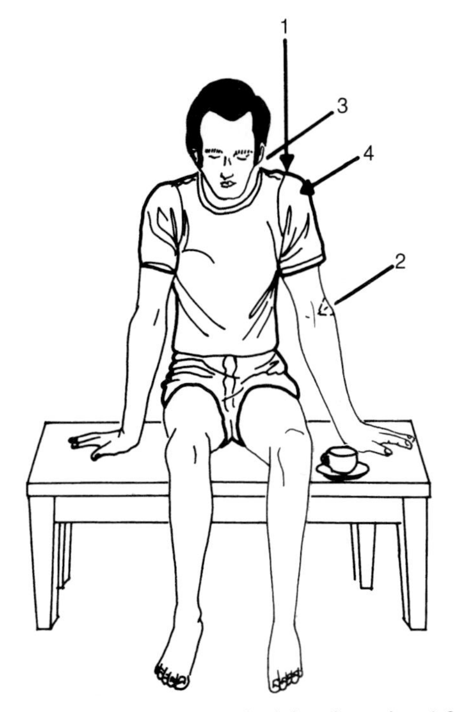

Fig. 19 Stabilizing in sitting. The helper uses both hands to give: 1 & 2, gentle pressure downwards from shoulder to hand with elbow support; 3, gentle pressure to the back of the head to give spinal extension with thrust through the arms; 4, gentle pressure laterally at the shoulder will finally maintain the position. Pressures should be built up slowly and withdrawn slowly.

pattern on an outwardly rotated shoulder. The PNF definition of approximation is 'the compression of a segment or extremity through the long axis'. The effect is to stimulate a muscular response and improve stability. Used in inhibiting patterns it is the quickest way to get the desired tone into the arm.

Figure 20 shows a compression technique. This is hard work for the physiotherapist if she is to maintain the pressure between the heel of the patient's hand and his scapula for any length of time. Stability in side-lying has been established. If an assistant is available, she may provide the counter-pressure through the scapula and outwardly rotated shoulder.

Note: If this manipulation gives pain, *stop at once* as you are doing something wrong. Check the shoulder position carefully. As illustrated in Figure 20, a little more outward rotation of the hand could be used to advantage.

Figure 21 shows the patient inhibiting his own arm. As soon as it is practicable, he should be taught the need for corrective positioning and how to take over the care of his own limbs. In this position, he is encouraged to begin trunk rolling patterns. As illustrated here, the physiotherapist is helping to stabilize the shoulder position while she also assists in mobilizing the lower trunk with hip rolling backwards and forwards.

Figures 7–19 represent some of the inhibiting positions and exercising patterns that are taught and used in the early days of rehabilitation. The aim has been to establish inhibiting patterns, to take care of the vital early shoulder care, to begin rolling from side to side, to stabilize in side-lying and to lead into transfer from bed to chair with the need to maintain inhibiting patterns when sitting out of bed and, finally, to establish sitting balance.

Figures 20 and 21 described above, show the beginning of mat work. To avoid repetition, the further development of mat work will be described in Chapter 4.

BUILDING ON DEVELOPMENT OF CONTROLLED MOVEMENT AS SEEN IN THE INFANT

The following points should be borne in mind:

1. Fetal movements are reflex movements and are called primitive, but these primitive movements are the predecessors of all purposeful, coordinated actions.

2. At birth, the first movements are still primitive: eye movements, head turning, kicking, finger grasp and so on.

In stroke rehabilitation, start rolling patterns by turning eyes and head in the direction of the roll. Where necessary the physiotherapist causes the patient's eyes to move in the direction of the roll (e.g. by clapping her hands) and the roll is encouraged to follow the eyes and the head.

3. A single primitive movement may trigger off a long chain of reflex actions,

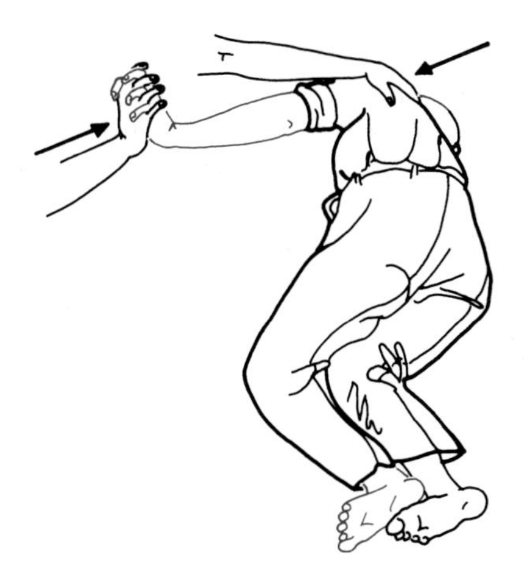

Fig. 20 The elderly patient usually takes longer to mobilize. Shoulder reached well forward, patient pushing (compression or weightbearing through the heel of the hand).

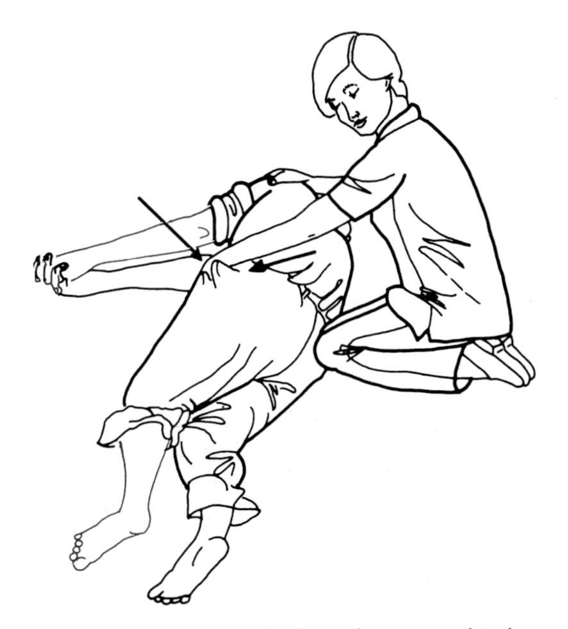

Fig. 21 Arm positioned, upper and lower trunk rotations are assisted.

for example, sucking leading to head tilting, head tilting to extending the arms, etc.

See the patient's body as a whole and guard against any unwanted chain reaction which, with the brain damage of stroke and consequent imbalance of muscle tone, may follow and increase unwanted antigravity tonal patterns.

4. With the passage of time the restless, primitive movements of the newborn

infant develop into controlled movement which can be performed deliberately or automatically.

Stroke rehabilitation, to be successful, depends on constant repetition of all therapeutic movements which work into inhibiting patterns.

5. Motor development in the infant is from head to foot in direction, that is from proximal to distal, or neck and shoulder before elbow and hand, trunk and hip before knee and foot.

Start with the trunk but, at the same time, maintain inhibiting patterns in the limbs.

6. As this motor development takes place the infant develops his postural reflex mechanism. Postural stability and controlled movements progress hand in hand; the outward and visible sign of inward and invisible reflex happenings, leading forward to the completion of the developing nervous system.

To recover postural stability and controlled movement, irradiation and the use of associated reactions to strengthen the weak muscles can be invaluable, provided strong and adequate control of antigravity tone can be maintained.

7. It is important to remember that motor development and sensory development proceed together.

Guided by these motor development patterns, stroke rehabilitation has a sound foundation on which to base a recovery programme. It begins with the patient in lying which gives the wide base, low centre of gravity and the sense of security that the patient needs. This makes it possible to follow a logical plan, with a reasoned approach to the problems presented by loss of normal muscle tone and consequently, loss of the postural reflex mechanism. At the same time sensory input will be given a reasonable boost.

ARM RECOVERY

Figure 22 illustrates some positions the child uses in his motor development sequence, i.e. five advancing positions in which he bears weight through his arms. This sequence suggests that as hemiplegia presents us with the especially difficult problem of arm recovery, we should attempt to increase greatly the time spent on exercise techniques such as the following, which mimic this developmental sequence:

1. Weightbearing on forearms with head lifted backwards, i.e. tonic neck extension.
2. Balanced over forearms, neck extension with rotation to the affected side.
3. Transfer of weight over to the affected side to free the sound arm.
4. Balancing weight on hands, elbow extension, correct use of tonic neck extension with rotation to the affected side, continues to increase extensor thrust through the affected arm.
5. Increasing the demand made in 4.

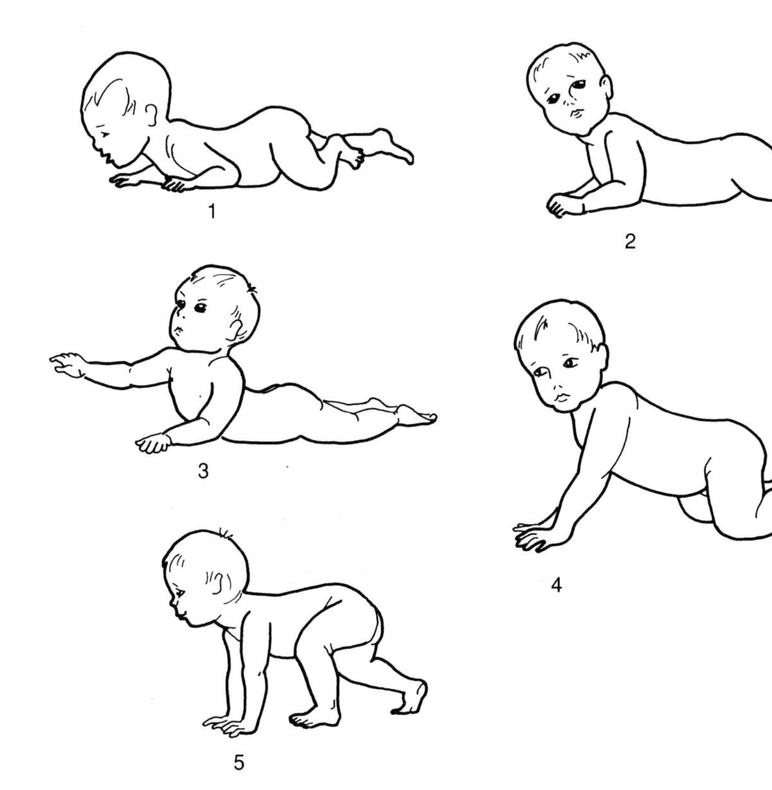

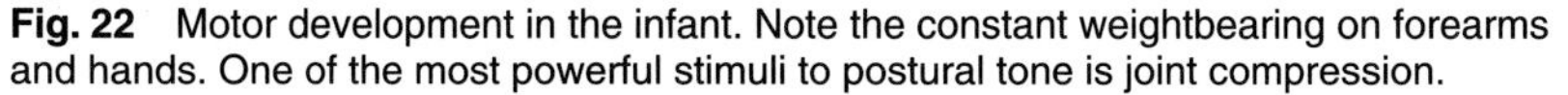

Fig. 22 Motor development in the infant. Note the constant weightbearing on forearms and hands. One of the most powerful stimuli to postural tone is joint compression.

FURTHER COMMENTS ON DEVELOPMENT OF CONTROLLED MOVEMENT IN THE INFANT

Base your exercise programme on developmental patterns.

1. The infant learns to roll. He repeats his new trick again and again. With constant repetition of this new movement, and because of the alterations in the position of his head in space and in relation to his trunk and extremities, postural and righting reflexes are called into action.

Note again the need for constant repetition. The affected arm is best controlled as illustrated in Figure 12.

2. Rolling from supine to prone becomes a controlled and functional movement and he rolls to prop on his forearms (Fig. 22, 2). He begins to extend and rotate his cervical spine (Fig. 22, 2).

Make full and correct use of tonic neck reflexes.

3. He extends his head in prone; he begins to extend his arms (Fig. 22, 3), and he begins to crawl on his forearms, dragging his legs.

Make every possible attempt to keep arm rehabilitation ahead of leg recovery.

4. He also learns to roll from supine to sitting; the more complicated equilibrium responses are developing.

Make correct use of these responses to produce the desired shifts in muscle tone; know and understand the levels of reflex activity.

5. Forearm crawling leads to pushing himself backward and he gets onto all fours.

Establish the crawling position whenever possible. Begin crawling exercise by rocking backwards and forwards over the hands (Fig. 22, 4).

6. Stabilized in the crawling position, and with rocking movements over his hands, he frees his primitive flexor grip and releases his hands for functional movement.

Only then can the stroke patient perform true functional movements of the hand which depend on restoration of normal muscle tone to allow fine precision movements to take place.

Note: If we take into account the constant use of weightbearing through arm and hand in this developmental sequence, it would suggest that the hemiplegic arm must be used in weight bearing in inhibiting patterns and possible modifications introduced as early as possible after the onset of a stroke. Do not use any manipulation which causes pain.

ROLLING

It will be expected that in applying this developmental sequence to the stroke patient, rolling will be used with constant repetition all through the treatment programme, beginning as early as is practical in the active exercise programme. This is because rolling is a functional activity and an exercise for the whole body. It mobilizes and strengthens the trunk, inhibiting extensor spasticity provided flexion patterns are used with the exception of the forearm and hand. It brings in righting reactions and equilibrium responses, and leads into recovery of standing balance.

So what of the forearm and hand? Again the patient must be taught to inhibit his own arm by using the arm position illustrated in Figure 12. In the early days of treatment, the therapist gives any necessary assistance and ensures that only trunk flexion patterns are used, combined with inhibiting arm care.

When the bridging position of the affected leg is thoroughly established the patient will be ready to begin unassisted rolling, but with supervision until total corrective rolling patterns can be easily performed with stability in resting positions. Rolling from side to side comes first followed by total rolling patterns over and over across an adequate floor space. Resting periods should be in side-lying.

STABILIZATION

In applying the developmental sequence to the stroke patient, as rehabilitation progresses, stability will be established in the following positions:

1. In side-lying (both sides).
2. In prone lying with forearm propping (forearms parallel). For the elderly patient where necessary the position is modified.
3. In the crawling position with forearm support, and with modification if necessary.
4. In the full crawling position. This may be modified for osteoarthritic knees!
5. In stand or high kneeling.
6. In standing.

Many elderly people can undertake these progressions without any modification.

Weight bearing on the forearms and on the hands should be accepted as a very necessary part of arm rehabilitation and must be done within the inhibiting pattern.

Stability in sitting, as already described (see Fig. 19), should be established as early as possible in the programme, with careful positioning of the affected limbs.

OTHER POINTS

Careful assessment may be made to establish the patient's developmental level. To begin rehabilitation practice at a higher developmental level will simply reinforce the unwanted compensatory movements which will then increase unwanted antigravity tone (e.g. attempting to establish standing balance with support given to the patient on his sound side).

For any therapist who argues against the use of neurodevelopmental therapy (NDT), it must make sense to set out to recover lost balance by using mat work. This gives a wide base and a low centre of gravity, removing the fear of falling and substituting a sense of security, in the ideal situation for the introduction of rolling patterns. To carry out the required rolling patterns is, in many ways, to mimic motor development patterns.

Taking into account the size and action of the two major antigravity muscles, latissimus dorsi and gluteus maximus, it would seem to be logical to mobilize the trunk into bilateral rotation, with outward rotation of the hemiplegic shoulder and inward rotation of the hemiplegic hip, using the movement patterns which oppose the action of these two muscles.

Added to this is the fact that, for a large majority of stroke patients, rehabilitation, if it is to lead to a high standard of recovery and to an equally high quality of life, may take many weeks to accomplish and will depend on exercise routines which the patient will be able to master and then use with very little help. In this way, provided inhibiting positions and patterns are maintained and used at all times, each patient may be given the maximum chance of reaching his full recovery potential.

POSTSCRIPT

In 1966 I moved into a senior post in an acute hospital and set up a stroke unit which included the nurses. Following the motor development of the infant, my application techniques were strongly influenced by the long and excellent tuition I had had earlier in proprioceptive neurological facilitation (PNF), but at the same time took care not to use patterns which took the hip or shoulder into the nonrecovery rotations.

Also my treatment programme followed the motor development I had observed in my own small son and other children, but with one exception: that a serious attempt was made to stay within the antigravity inhibiting patterns already described. Irradiation and the use of associated reactions to increase diverted tonal overflow into inhibiting patterns were not acceptable unless strong and adequate control of antigravity tone was maintained. Every effort was made to shift antigravity tone into the opposing low tonal patterns.

I directed and worked with this rehabilitation unit for 3 years and carefully assessed the clinical results. All patients with completed strokes who were judged ready for rehabilitation by the senior physician were included in the clinical trial. All had been admitted to the hospital on day 1 of the onset of the stroke. Our main item of equipment was a very large floor mat.

The rehabilitation results were very satisfactory, except for recovery of a useful arm. We began to expect to finish with a balanced trunk and a good walking gait, but arm recovery was very disappointing. Developing hypertonicity in the hemiplegic arm had not been successfully inhibited; hypotonicity did not allow sufficient stability to make it possible to undertake the ambitious advancing programme that had been planned and, added to this, eventually spasticity was usually seen to begin creeping into the fingers.

However, continuing to work in the same unit for a further 5 years, we reversed our results in arm rehabilitation. I had found a suitable method to control tonal flow in the hemiplegic arm. The answer was the use of a plastic inflatable splint which had been developed as a tool to be used in first aid ambulance care when transporting accident cases with fractured arms. Here was the ideal tool to stabilize limbs in inhibiting patterns while rehabilitation was undertaken.

Chapter 4 presents the use of inflatable splints in a realistic approach to the brain damage of stroke.

REFERENCES

Adler S S, Beckers D, Buck M 1993 PNF in practice: an illustrated guide. Springer-Verlag, Berlin

Johnston T B, Davies D V, Davies F 1958 Gray's anatomy, 32nd edn. Longman, London

Knott M, Voss D 1968 Proprioceptive neuromuscular facilitation: patterns and techniques. Harper and Row, New York

McGlown D 1990 Developmental reflexive rehabilitation. Taylor and Francis, London

4

THE USE OF PRESSURE SPLINTS

INTRODUCTION

The physiotherapist and the nurse, must use careful positioning to act as the inhibiting influence on hypertonic motor neurones until the postural reflex mechanism is re-established, or until the static reflexes once more become integrated into controlled movement. This happens when normal inhibiting influences have been restored. In other words, at all times, correct positioning is used to replace the inhibiting influence from cortical level that is missing. Or, corrective positioning is used to influence the distribution of the patient's muscle tone at all times while rehabilitation is undertaken.

It is frequently possible to teach a family member to undertake this important duty. As much of the rehabilitation programme may be undertaken in the home, such involvement is more than helpful. The family member or home carer should be carefully taught the reason for the patient's spasticity problem and, therefore, the vital need to use positioning to prevent the build-up of spasticity which may soon reach crippling proportions. It is not difficult to put the information into lay language and, with understanding, the carer can often become dedicated to the patient's need.

However, even with the greatest possible care in the specialized stroke unit, it had become very clear that careful positioning and the use of inhibiting patterns had not been enough to prevent the development of spasticity in the hemiplegic arm. Remembering that associated reactions occur with all attempted movements to give a widespread increase in spasticity in the affected limbs if the latter are not inhibited, why should arm rehabilitation fail when this was not the case in the rest of the body? Total inhibiting patterns for hemiplegic disability are flexion patterns except for the forearm and hand. Here the limb must be inhibited by maintaining and working into extension patterns, i.e. the opposite pattern to the rest of the body. This was probably the greatest contributing factor to failure to recover a working hand with fine precision movements and skilled function.

Considering these facts, the obvious and logical conclusion was that a more effective way of controlling antigravity tone in the forearm and hand must be found. Associated reactions and all overflow of tone must be diverted into extension patterns. Rigid splints had been rejected. To attempt to hold the forearm in extension with a rigid splint fastened to the flexor aspect of the elbow, wrist and fingers resulted in an increase of unwanted flexor tone, as the arm flexed ever harder against this rigid support. Would the inflatable splint answer the problem?

APPLYING THE INFLATABLE PRESSURE SPLINT TO THE ARM

Figure 23 illustrates the inflatable pressure splint for the arm. It is used to stabilize the hemiplegic arm, maintaining the inhibiting forearm pattern of extension of the elbow, wrist and fingers. The splint is applied with the patient lying on his back, knees flexed as in Figure 8. To complete the required inhibiting pattern a small pillow under the shoulders will give mild neck extension and the patient's head should be rotated towards the affected side. The three stages used for easy application are shown in Figure 23.

Stage A

1. Close the zip fastener.
2. Pull the splint onto your own arm and take a handshake grasp of the patient's affected hand.
3. Rotate the shoulder outwards, extend the elbow and pull the splint onto the patient's positioned arm.

Stage B

1. Maintain the correct hand position, making sure that the thumb is fully abducted.
2. Inflate the splint by mouth. The length of the inflation tube makes it possible to hold the tube with your teeth leaving two hands free to manage the splint. Warm air from the lungs warms and moulds the inner sleeve to the arm giving all over even pressure with no danger of constriction. Using the human lungs means that the splint should not be overinflated, but it must be firmly applied with a pressure of 38–40 mmHg. The PVC splint is

transparent and the position of the limb inside is clearly visible, and should always be checked. The fingertips must be well back from the open end and a cotton sleeve should be worn next to the patient's skin to prevent a sweat rash. Never allow the patient to sit out in the sun while wearing the splint.

Stage C

1. The air that has been blown in by mouth inflates the space between inner and outer sleeves leaving the arm well cushioned and maintained in the inhibiting pattern. As suggested above, the splint is easiest to apply with the patient lying in supine, positioned to assist extensor tone in the forearm, and remembering to inhibit extensor tone in the rest of the body.
2. If the splint is to be applied with the patient in sitting, then he should lean back in his chair, tilt his head backward and rotate it towards his affected side.

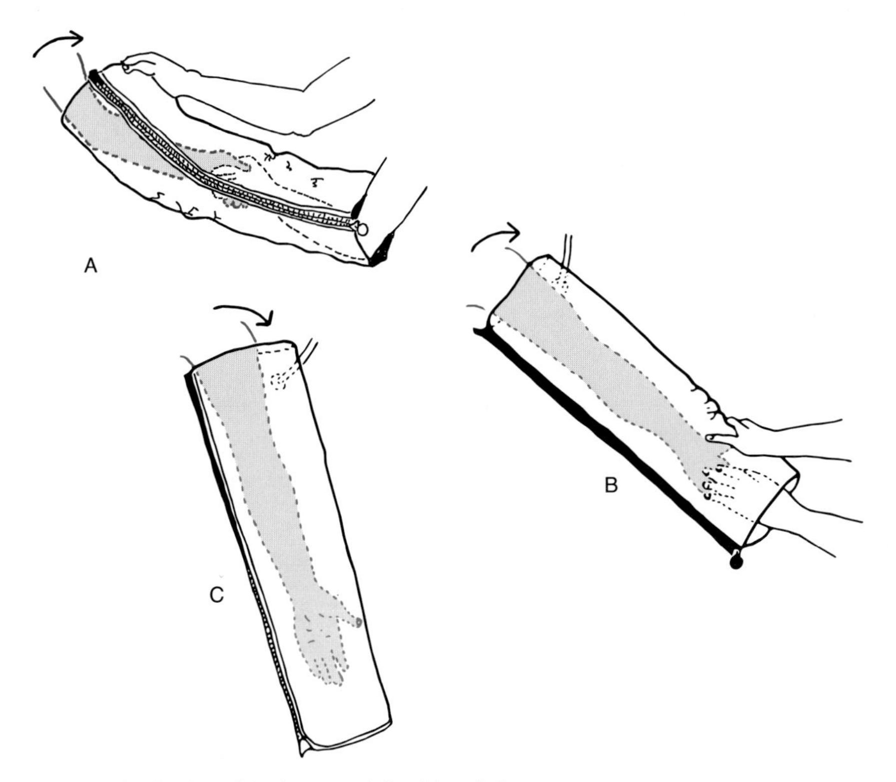

Fig. 23 Application of the long arm inflatable splint.

THE SHOULDER

Figure 24 serves as a reminder that at no time should the importance of outward rotation of the shoulder be forgotten. Even given the ever present need to inhibit the dominant antigravity tonal pattern of latissimus dorsi, it should be noted that this is not the only reason for the urgent need to maintain this shoulder pattern.

THE AGONY SHOULDER

The agony shoulder of the stroke patient is an all too frequent development after the onset of a stroke. It is not difficult to prevent this unnecessary distress provided the cause is understood and, where there is understanding, preventive measures will be taken.

So why does the shoulder joint give trouble? The following factors are involved:

1. It is a lax joint at the best of times.
2. It is dependent on the normal plane of the joint between scapula and humerus.
3. It is dependent on a normal supraspinatus muscle.
4. It is dependent on the rotator cuff ligament.
5. It is dependent on a mobile scapula.

After a stroke all the above factors may be involved.

Hemiplegic shoulder pain occurs because of:

1. the altered plane of the joint
2. the muscle weakness
3. a lax ligament
4. an immobile scapula.

The result is:

1. impinging of bone surfaces between humerus and scapula
2. pinching of the rotator cuff
3. damage to the supraspinatus.

Damage occurs in these situations:

1. If the patient is rolled over onto a disabled shoulder which is trapped below his body weight in inward rotation.

2. If the patient is pulled up the bed by an inwardly rotated shoulder.

3. If the patient is assisted in any way by pulling on or weightbearing through an inwardly rotated shoulder.

4. If the patient's upper trunk and shoulder, particularly the scapula, are not therapeutically treated to establish and maintain upper trunk and scapula mobility.

5. If measures are not taken to restore shoulder stability.

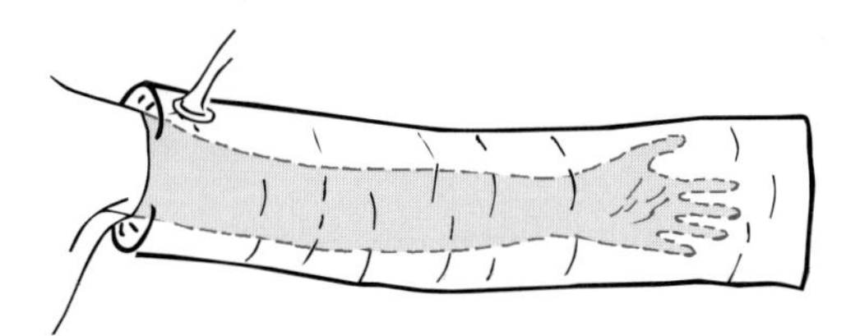

Fig. 24 Outward rotation of the shoulder, with the splint inhibiting flexor spasticity of forearm and hand.

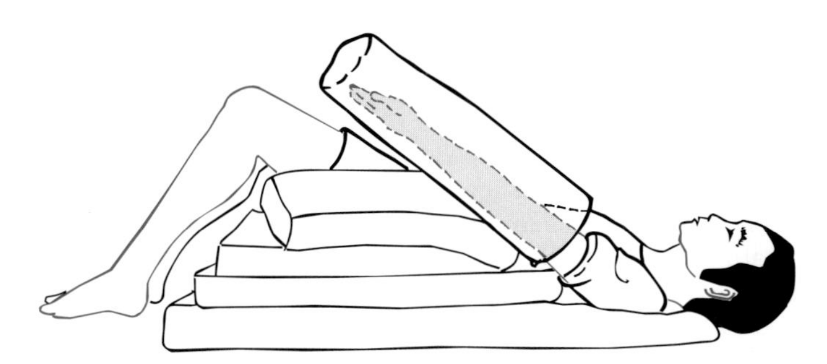

Fig. 25 Resting position in inhibiting, or recovery, pattern.

It will be found that, properly applied, the inflatable splint greatly assists shoulder treatment.

Figure 25 illustrates the best resting position to be used when lying on the back is required at any stage of treatment.

Rehabilitation for the stroke patient starts with the trunk; the upper trunk includes the shoulder and, from the earliest days, care of the shoulder should be seen as a priority. Furthermore, you cannot stabilize a trunk on an unstable arm. The inflatable splint stabilizes the arm.

TREATMENT FOR THE SHOULDER JOINT

The following points should be noted:

1. All treatment should be undertaken with the long arm splint in place to divert all overflow of tone into the inhibiting pattern for elbow, wrist and fingers.

2. With application of the full arm splint and positioning as in Figure 25, an immediate relaxation of shoulder muscles can be seen. Note that the splint does not control the shoulder but the clear plastic material of the splint makes it possible to see the position of the enclosed limb. To maintain the correct shoulder position *the thumb should always point outward, away from the body.*

3. Mobilize the upper trunk. Remember that latissimus dorsi has extensive origins in the trunk and spasticity in this area may occur fairly rapidly after

the onset of a stroke, giving side flexion with shortening of the trunk and retraction with inward rotation of the shoulder.

4. Keep the scapula mobile so that free movement allows it to slide round the chest wall.

5. Therapists work to mobilize and maintain the necessary outward rotation of the shoulder.

6. Nurses must always use and maintain this shoulder pattern of outward rotation in their care of the patient. Do physiotherapists teach this where necessary? If not, why not? All members of any team, hospital- or home-based, should understand this vital need.

7. Get tone into the shoulder as quickly as possible by giving compression through the outwardly rotated shoulder. If it hurts, you are doing something wrong. Make sure the shoulder is in outward rotation and there is firm support behind the scapula.

8. Between physiotherapy sessions, supply a shoulder support where it may be felt to be necessary (not a sling which will rotate the shoulder into inward rotation across the front of the body), but make sure it truly maintains the vital outward rotation. A broad crepe bandage applied in a figure-of-eight with the crossover at the back and going under alternate axillae, holding a firm supporting pad under the affected shoulder and bracing both shoulders back, can give a very satisfactory support. For comfort and to help bring the shoulders level, a smaller pad may be used under the sound shoulder. If the patient has no objection the bandage may be applied on top of clothing where it is seen as a reminder to all helpers that the shoulder must be handled with great care.

9. Use advancing weightbearing techniques to get tone into the shoulder, e.g. sitting as in Figure 19 but supporting the affected arm with the inflatable splint. The quickest way to get tone into a limb is to bear weight through the limb. Always make sure the limb is used in this way, while maintaining the inhibiting pattern; if not there is a real danger of increasing the unwanted antigravity tone. Check the weightbearing base (Fig. 26).

SUBLUXATION OF THE SHOULDER

There are other problems with the hemiplegic shoulder which should be taken into account in the early days of rehabilitation. Subluxation of the shoulder is not uncommon.

This should not be a problem if handled correctly.

1. Use a long arm pressure splint, and give compression with the shoulder joint in outward rotation.

2. Maintaining the vital outward rotation of the shoulder, and giving stability to the elbow, wrist and fingers in extension with the support of the inflated splint, use the weightbearing techniques suggested above.

3. Note that many physiotherapists worry unnecessarily about subluxation of the affected shoulder in the stroke patient. The flaccid or hypotonic hanging arm will sublux but this is not a reason for undue concern, provided careful,

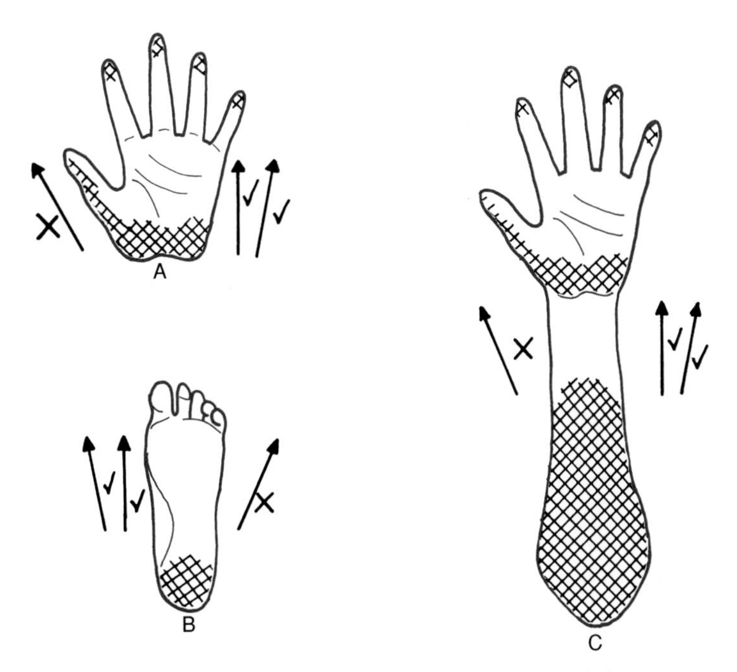

Fig. 26 Weightbearing over a correctly positioned base, seen from below. A. The heel of the hand. B. The heel of the foot. C. The forearm and hand.

correct handling is undertaken on the lines already suggested. Without adequate stabilizing support, because of the mechanical position of the scapula with the glenoid cavity, subluxation follows. Adequate stabilizing support is supplied by the pressure splint.

4. To sum up, in the early days after onset of the stroke, if the patient is correctly handled, and this includes the maintenance of a free scapula, weightbearing through a correctly positioned shoulder will replace the mechanical stability of the shoulder joint.

5. Pain has nothing to do with subluxation; pain is associated with strained and damaged muscles and ligaments, resulting from wrong positioning and bad lifting. It is associated with an immobile scapula and with spasticity and contractures. Unless preventative measures are taken these problems can develop all too quickly. The physiotherapist may be left to deal with the effects of neglect and bad handling, and she must release the scapula before she can make any sort of beginning to re-educate controlled movement in the shoulder.

SHOULDER AND ARM PROBLEMS

The use of the pressure splint and pressure techniques introduced early in the rehabilitation programme will prevent serious problems from developing, and will also go a long way towards solving the problems that may have to be faced if early treatment has not been possible. To be forewarned is to be forearmed and this would seem to be the place to present other shoulder and arm problems that may have to be dealt with.

THE STIFF PAINFUL SHOULDER

The physiotherapist may inherit this problem if she takes on a patient for late treatment.

1. There is usually spasticity in the trunk.
2. Start with the trunk, but first apply a long arm splint.
3. Position the patient, lying on his sound side as in Figure 9 but have him lying over a pillow to elongate the trunk on his affected side. Start with a rest period in this position.
4. Same position: separately teach upper and lower trunk rotations. Start with passive mobilization, progress to active assisted work and then on to active work (Fig. 27).
5. Same position: manually mobilize the scapula with one hand while supporting the splinted arm with the other hand. Deep frictions round the posterior scapular border will be useful and a comfortable oil massage may be given to the whole area.
6. Same position: trunk rolling in opposite rotations.
7. Roll the patient onto his back with his legs in the crook position (as for bridging), support the splinted arm in elevation with outward rotation, and mobilize the shoulder, using your free hand to support the scapula and to assist in mobilizing the shoulder in protraction.
8. Roll back into the side-lying position and mobilize the shoulder by assisting the splinted arm in a sawing movement across the pillows which are supporting the arm.

THE FLACCID HYPOTONIC LIMB

The hypotonic arm with greatly reduced muscle tone resulting in the heavy 'rag-doll' limb of flaccid paralysis is possibly the most difficult problem to be faced. It can so easily continue into long-term flaccidity (or hypotonus) where the arm becomes a useless appendage hanging at the patient's side. To get tone into the arm, weightbearing techniques must be used. However, again, the long arm inflatable splint has much to offer.

1. Apply the long arm splint.
2. Use all possible weightbearing techniques but keep the shoulder in outward rotation.
3. There is usually a need to substantially increase sensory input. Again pressure from the splint which is used in altering positions and movements will increase this.
4. Is there a need to increase sensory input to stimulate muscular proprio-

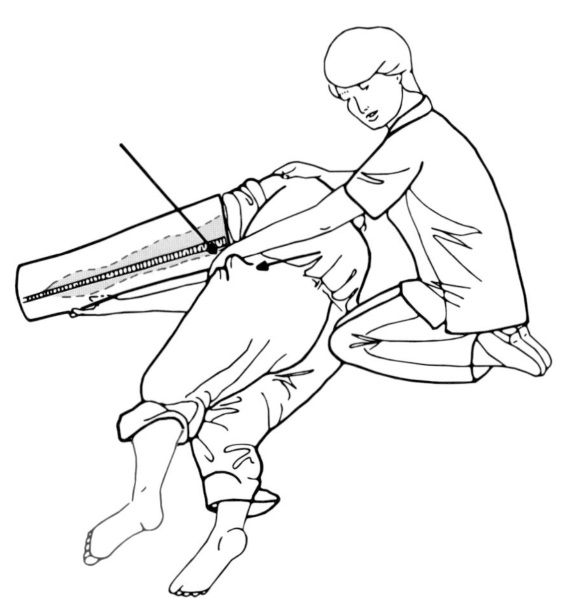

Fig. 27 The pressure splint maintains the inhibiting arm pattern while trunk rotations are assisted.

ceptors? Could this be done by introducing a mechanical pump? This later became a question which had to be answered.

5. Use compression techniques to stimulate joint proprioceptors.
6. Where available the tilt table can be introduced early in the programme to great advantage, with arm weightbearing included, making prolonged weightbearing possible. (Take care of the leg pattern by using a small roll behind the knees to maintain enough knee flexion to break the extension pattern, and position feet so that weight goes through the heels.)
7. Remember that flexor spasticity may develop even in the formerly flaccid arm if inhibiting patterns are not carefully maintained at all times. Carefully assess your patient's progress.
8. Tapping and pounding can be useful. Also *quick* ice treatment may have a place here.

Treatment on these lines will often give very satisfactory results.

OEDEMA OF THE HAND

This occurs when the hemiplegic arm has not been carefully positioned and has been allowed to hang down at the patient's side giving gravitational oedema. This is not a problem if careful positioning and pressure techniques have been used. However, if it occurs, as may be the case where late treatment is offered, it should be dealt with immediately.

1. Use pressure splints for treatment sessions and give passive manipulations with the full arm splint supporting the limb as in Figure 25. For example, give wrist flexion and extension following the initial resting position.
2. Use positioning at all times and include positioning with elevation.
3. Should intermittent pressure be used? (Note point 4 in the section above on the flaccid hypotonic limb.) Again this was considered as a question that had to be answered. There were certain contraindications.
4. Use weightbearing exercise with long arm pressure splint support in inhibiting patterns as soon as the oedema is under control.
5. Wherever possible, hand over the care of his own limb to the patient himself. At first, constantly remind him to position his own arm.
6. Sitting in a chair will begin early in this programme and so, early on it is necessary to supply a suitable arm rest, for example, a gutter arm rest on the arm of the chair. This is a necessity for all arm rehabilitation. In the early days a drip stand and a roller towel can be used to give good arm support. The drip stand is placed on the patient's affected side and the towel adjusted to support the arm in elevation.

PREVENTION AND TREATMENT

Shoulder and arm problems that must be faced have perhaps been placed out of context here. However, this has been done with the suggestion that early understanding of the problems will result in early introduction of the preventative measures that should be taken. None of these problems needs to happen. Preventative treatment occurs quite naturally if correct rehabilitation practices are followed.

For example, as already mentioned, never roll a stroke patient onto his affected side with his affected shoulder trapped below his body in inward rotation. The resulting damage to the shoulder will lead to the agony shoulder syndrome which will effectively put an end to rehabilitation hopes. The patient will nurse the affected arm with his forearm supported across his body, and the shoulder in inward rotation. Pain will build up spasticity and the patient will not allow anyone near him.

In this case the physiotherapist will need to use all her skill and care to reassure and treat the patient with the use of heat, in some cases ice, massage and relaxation until she begins gently to mobilize the trunk and the shoulder (into outward rotation). With the application of the long arm inflatable pressure splint there is a quite noticeable relaxation of shoulder girdle muscles. The agony shoulder in the stroke patient ought not to occur.

THE USE OF THE LONG ARM SPLINT

The validity of any rehabilitation concept for the treatment of stroke, as already said, must be judged by the success or failure of the results obtained in the clinical field. With the introduction of the long arm pressure splint into treatment practices, success seemed at once to be within easy reach. However, subjective evidence was not enough; scientific evidence was not at first forthcoming and it took 10 years of clinical practice, including the development of a series of splints and laboratory tests, to convince the sceptics that here was a treatment concept which ought to be explored.

REASONS FOR USING THE PRESSURE SPLINT

Early development of the pressure splint programme was built on the use of neuromotor development patterns, incorporating pressure splints where necessary to inhibit unwanted excessive antigravity tone. The stability of sustained posture is necessary for rehabilitation, and because of the imbalance of muscle tone, the stroke patient lacks stability. Added to this, you cannot stabilize the trunk on unstable limbs. There seemed to be five good reasons for using the pressure splint for the hemiplegic arm:

1. to stabilize the limb
2. to inhibit antigravity tone
3. to control associated reactions
4. to increase sensory input
5. to assist early weightbearing.

The splint is applied as described on pp. 50–51.

As already suggested, to start any stroke patient's rehabilitation above his developmental level is to reinforce compensatory movement and, with the brain damage of stroke, this will not work. Because of the loss of normal muscle tone, a large majority of these patients must start rehabilitation as the human infant starts, i.e. with rotational patterns. For the stroke patient this means trunk into bilateral rotation, shoulder into outward rotation, hip into inward rotation.

Because of the loss of normal postural tone and the consequent loss of the normal postural reflex mechanism, flexion patterns are used to inhibit antigravity tone in the whole body except for the forearm and hand; here an outside inhibiting force must be added to divert tonal flow into extension in this area. All those who care for the stroke patient must provide the missing inhibitory influence. The introduction of the pressure splint gave new hope to the possible recovery of motor function in the forearm and hand. Mat work becomes essential.

WEIGHTBEARING

Figure 28 shows compression through the heel of the hand to a shoulder in outward rotation with protraction, putting tone into the shoulder using the full inhibiting pattern. In the acute unit, with early treatment and the introduction of the pressure splint for the arm, many of the shoulder problems did not occur, or, if there was a problem it was possible to deal with it. For example, compression techniques to put tone into the subluxed shoulder were easy to apply with the shoulder-to-hand inhibiting pattern fully maintained as in Figure 28. Again, this must be performed with the shoulder in outward rotation, while a second therapist gives supporting pressure over the scapula.

Compression, approximation and weightbearing all have the same meaning: they are techniques which put weight through the length of a limb, an essential feature of all worthwhile treatment. The pressure splint is used to maintain the essential inhibiting pattern and to stimulate and produce the same effects as weightbearing, giving postural fixation with sensory stimulation, allowing the necessary weightbearing to be undertaken. As illustrated here, approximation from the heel of the hand to the shoulder is given with counterpressure from the outwardly rotated shoulder.

Weightbearing bases must always be correct. Referring back, Figure 26 illustrates the correct weightbearing bases used to inhibit antigravity tone. It should be noted that here you are looking at the weightbearing bases from below. The hatched areas show the surface areas where most weight should be transmitted.

Figure 26A, showing weightbearing through the hand, illustrates the need to place the hand pointing straight forward or outwardly to ensure that the shoulder joint above is maintained in outward rotation. This will not increase unwanted antigravity tone and will have a positive effect on the opposing weak tonal pattern.

This is an appropriate place to introduce the correct weightbearing base in the foot (Fig. 26B). Here weight must be transmitted through the heel, with the foot pointing straight forward or into moderate inward rotation, and not through the front of an outwardly rotated foot. This is to ensure that gluteus maximus is not contributing to a strong antigravity thrust.

Figure 26C shows weightbearing through the forearm and hand. The forearm points straight forward or into outward rotation, again to make sure the shoulder joint is not allowed to bear weight in the antigravity pattern of inward rotation.

By observing these simple rules, an important factor in the recovery of normal movement has been taken into account in the use of the pressure splint to support the treatment programme and is an integral part of the basic concept.

THE PLACING RESPONSE

Figure 29 shows an important stage in arm rehabilitation which must not be neglected. It is the need to work towards recovery of a placing response.

'Placing' is a term that ought to be understood. The normal human being has the ability to 'place' a limb. This means he can maintain a limb in space in any position. The ability to do this may be lost where there is a change in muscle tone; for example, the stroke patient's limb will usually drift into the dominant reflex pattern, i.e. spasticity.

In Figure 29 the patient has not yet fully recovered a placing response in the shoulder. Here the patient attempts to hold his arm in elevation and to increase protraction while the therapist helps to maintain the necessary outward rotation. All possible exercise techniques to increase shouldertone in the inhibiting pattern must be used and, of these, corrective weight bearing is the most important. There is a vital need to establish a placing response in the hemiplegic shoulder as early as possible in the recovery programme. Without the support of the pressure splint this is not possible.

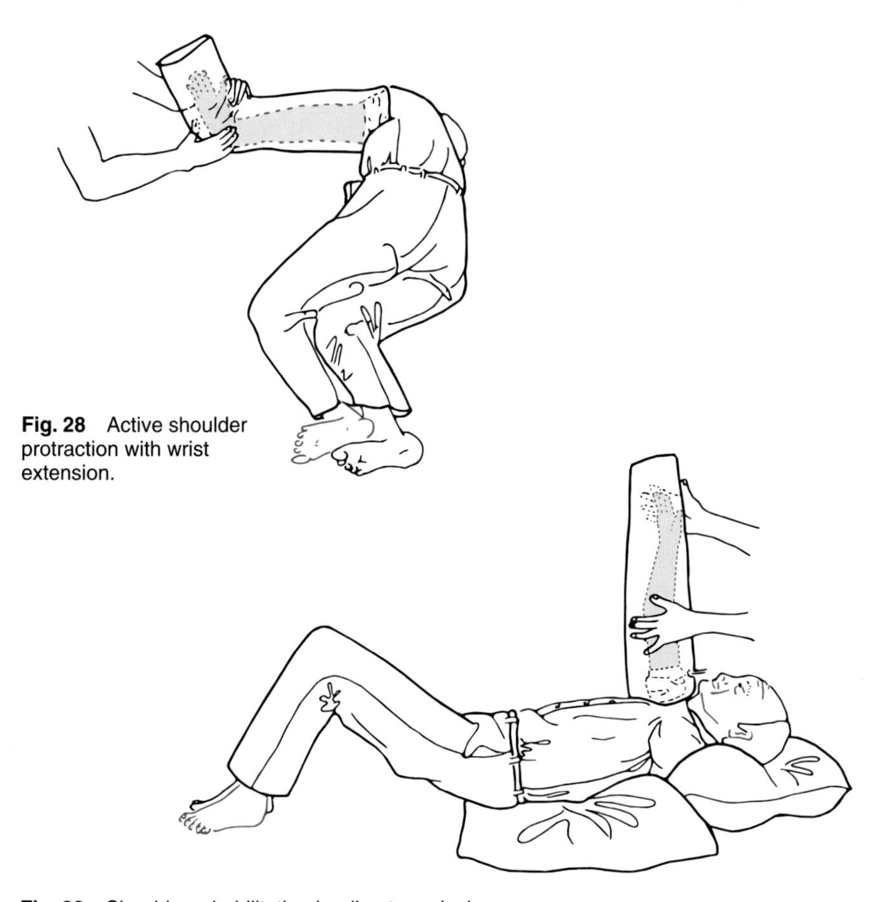

Fig. 28 Active shoulder protraction with wrist extension.

Fig. 29 Shoulder rehabilitation leading to a placing response.

TREATMENT RESULTS

Five years of practice, using the long arm pressure splint in the acute hospital, in many cases, led to most satisfactory treatment results, with arm rehabilitation advancing ahead of leg recovery, but the final outcome also presented a good walking gait with a firm heel strike.

It has to be remembered that the hospital admitted patients on day 1 of the onset of the stroke and even the unconscious patient was carefully positioned. There was no chance of damage to the affected shoulder by turning the patient into the no-win position of lying on a shoulder which was trapped below his body. The full cooperation of the nursing staff was necessary here.

Progress continued through the specialized physiotherapy unit, for all survivors, and continued on into outpatient care provided by the same unit. Careful inhibiting positions and patterns were used at all times and motor development patterns, as taught by Norman Dott (see Ch. 2), were used. Developing deformities were held at a minimum, e.g. the development of spasticity. The overall average length of time with this specialised care was 4 months. Perhaps it was the high rate of success achieved in this unit which gave a feeling of euphoria and a confident hope that here was a treatment concept which would surely make it possible for all stroke survivors to reach a high quality of life.

However, there were many difficulties ahead. At the present time many hospitals do not want specialized units. Both money and staff are scarce, but how does this balance out with the cost of the long-term care that is necessary for many post-stroke patients?

APPLYING THE TECHNIQUES TO LONG-TERM STROKE VICTIMS

Travelling round the world it was all too easy to find stroke patients with severe residual problems, prisoners in their own spasticity, walking with a marked hemiplegic gait, if they walked at all, and the affected arm a useless appendage held rigidly in the spasticity pattern.

It was time to move into the long-term hospital. Here stroke victims (who had failed to rehabilitate elsewhere and were unable to return to living in the community because of severe deformities) were expected to live out the remainder of their days in long-term care. Would it be possible at this late stage with the help of this more enlightened approach, and with the help of pressure techniques, to reverse deformities and lead back to a reasonable quality of life in the community?

Observing and carefully assessing the senior citizens in the long-term hospital was interesting and rewarding. Sitting balance was poor in most cases. Stability of the head, neck and upper trunk was often lacking and stability in side-lying often poor. Trunk rotation was poor or totally lacking, particularly when attempting to roll to the sound side which called for initiation from the weak side. In most cases the ability to bridge had not been taught; patients who fail to bridge do not achieve a good walking gait. In any attempt to restore motor recovery to a sufficiently high standard for the individual patient to return to the community with an acceptable quality of life, central stability with gross motor performance had to be achieved first.

Figures 30 and 31 relate child development stages to the patient's progress. In the acute hospital, with the pressure splint routine added to the recovery programme at the appropriate time, it had been quite possible in most cases to go ahead with motor developmental patterns. Would this still apply in the geriatric field with late treatment where deformities had already developed? In the acute hospital all age groups had been included, and all through the treatment programme the aim was to achieve useful recovery in the hemiplegic trunk, arm and leg. Inhibitory positioning and motor development patterns were used at all times, for example when standing and walking.

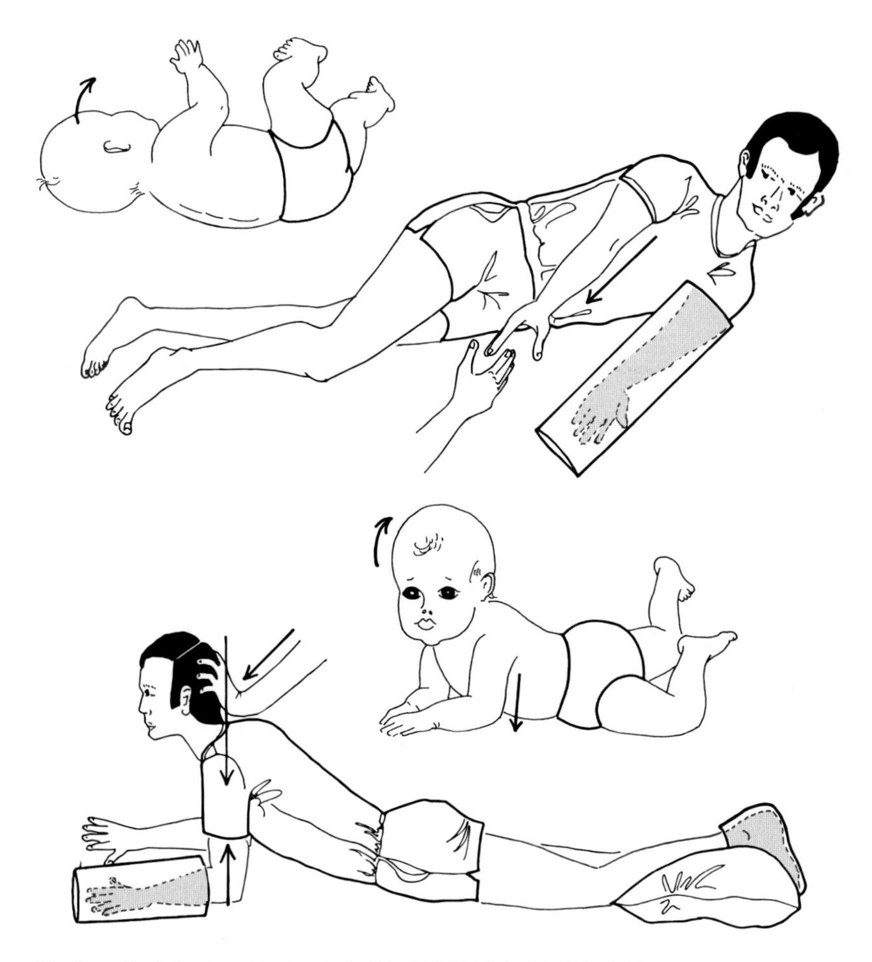

Fig. 30 Sustained pressure splints in training motor development.

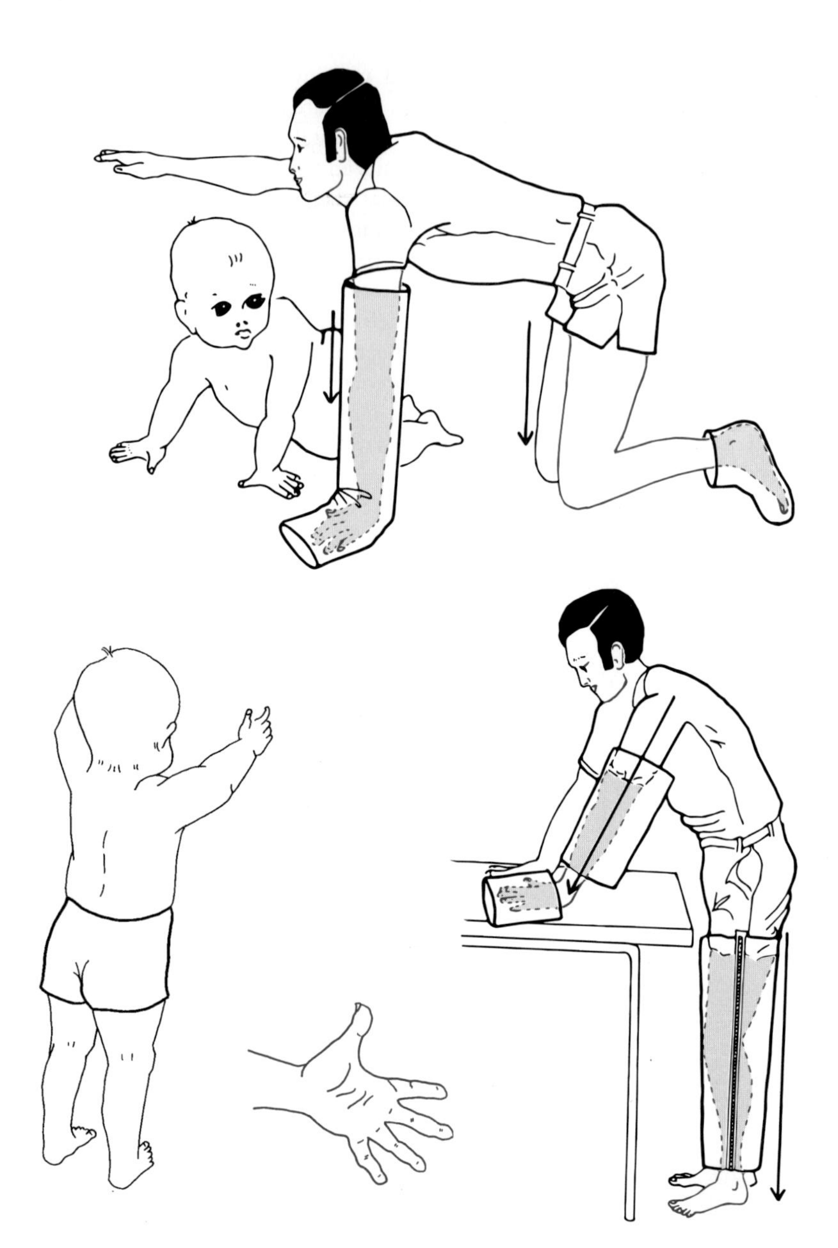

Fig. 31 More advanced training.

Figure 32 gives an example of the care taken when encouraging recovery of a good walking gait and it also serves as a reminder that all handling of the patient is approached from the affected side, using inhibiting patterns. Working from the patient's unaffected side would reinforce compensatory movement and destroy any hope of a return to normal movement. With the same line of thinking in the long-term hospital, with patients who had failed to rehabilitate elsewhere and who had already developed severe rehabilitation problems, it soon became evident that here was the ideal clinical setting in which to search for therapy skills which would address the problems related to long-standing spasticity, sensory loss, loss of the memory of normal movement and so on.

Again it was vital to start treatment at each patient's developmental level. To start above this level reinforced compensatory movement and put an end to any hope of recovery of normal movement. The state of each patient's muscle tone had to be very carefully assessed and it was very quickly established that the need in most cases was to start rehabilitation right back at the beginning using mat work, mobilizing the trunk into rotational patterns, reducing spasticity in the trunk, shoulder and hip and mobilizing the shoulder into outward rotation with protraction. The arm splint was invaluable and led to the development of a series of inflatable splints, each new splint designed to meet the needs of problem solving.

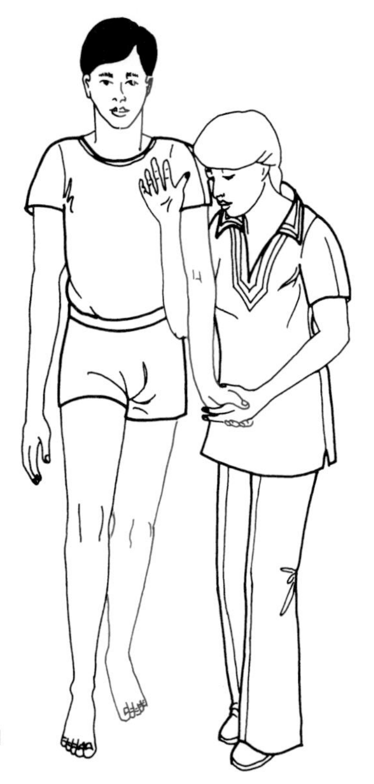

Fig. 32 Use inhibiting patterns and handle on the affected side.

NOTES ON THE USE OF PRESSURE SPLINTS

1. These splints, made of a unique and specially developed PVC sheeting, were designed by the author for the treatment of stroke and have been developed as the 'URIAS Stroke Rehabilitation Pressure Splints' by Palma-Plast.
2. The splints must be orally inflated; warm air from the lungs ensures a perfect fit, moulding the splint to the patient's limb to give all over even pressure. Lung pressure will not cause tissue damage to the patient, but athletes, players of the bagpipes and all who have above average lung capacity beware: *do not inflate to pressures over 40 mmHg*. If in doubt, test your pressure with a manometer.
3. A thin cotton sleeve should cover the patient's limb while the splint is in use, as a protection against sweat rash.
4. The splint should not be worn in direct sunlight. This would lead to excessive sweating, and strong sunlight through the plastic is liable to produce severe burns of the skin.
5. The splint should not be left on the limb for more than 1 hour at a time, but may be taken off and reapplied if longer time is required. It is often taken off and reapplied several times in the course of a treatment session.
6. When not in use the splint should not be folded but should lie flat or be hung up so that the inflation tube hangs downward to prevent strain at the junction between splint and tube.

These splints are now available for stroke treatment:

1. the long arm splint, in two lengths, 80 cm and 70 cm
2. the half-arm splint for use below the elbow
3. the foot splint
4. the elbow splint
5. the hand splint, in two lengths, 20 cm (8 inch) and 30 cm (12 inch)
6. the leg gaiter, in two lengths, 70 cm, average length, and 60 cm for the shorter leg.

THE LONG ARM SPLINT

This, probably the most useful and important splint, has already been introduced (see Fig. 23). It is important because without it it is not possible to maintain the vital inhibiting pattern of extension in the forearm, and to divert associated reactions into this extension pattern for more than brief spells and short exercise sessions. Without the arm splint, treatment is not dynamic enough to give satisfactory results.

By contrast it is considerably less difficult to maintain the necessary inhibitory patterns in the rest of the body because they are flexion patterns. Much of the patient's time is spent in the flexion pattern of sitting. However, introducing pressure splint control to tonal patterns in the rest of the body solves more problems and gives quicker treatment results.

THE HALF-ARM SPLINT

Method of application

This is applied below the elbow, leaving the elbow joint free for movement. The zip fastener is positioned on the side of the small finger along the border of the ulna. The wrist, fingers and thumb are positioned as in the long arm splint.

Use

1. To continue to control tonal distribution as rehabilitation progresses.
2. The patient is able early, to establish the prone position with forearm weightbearing with this splint as an aid. Forearms must be parallel.
3. In this prone position the therapist encourages weight shifts through the splinted forearm to increase shoulder stability.
4. The essential rehabilitation of elbow movements is achieved while the forearm inhibiting pattern is maintained.
5. In particular, the retraining of a strong triceps muscle is more easily obtained.

THE FOOT SPLINT

Method of application

This small boot must be applied with the patient's heel right back into the heel of the splint, making an angle of 90° in the ankle joint. It is easiest to apply with the patient lying supine and the therapist supporting the leg in the full inhibiting flexion position (pressure through the heel and inward rotation of the hip to reduce the extensor thrust in the leg). If this is wrongly applied, with the resulting pressure through the front of the sole of the foot, unwanted antigravity tone is increased.

Use

1. To assist in breaking up the antigravity extensor pattern in the leg and to maintain the inhibiting position of the foot.
2. To support the flaccid ankle where necessary, but note that this is not a splint for use in standing.

THE ELBOW SPLINT

Method of application

This is a short square splint applied to cover the elbow joint with an equal length of splint above and below this joint. Inflate with the zip running down the anterior aspect of the arm. As you inflate, grasp the fabric of the splint behind the elbow and allow this area to inflate last to give firm extensor support.

Use

1. To assist in elbow stability during exercises involving weightbearing through a correctly positioned hand, for example, weight bearing on hands and knees.
2. Used in conjunction with the hand splint.

THE HAND SPLINT

Method of application

This is a small double chamber splint applied with the hand in the inhibiting pattern with fingers in extension and the thumb abducted.

The chamber over the posterior aspect of the hand is inflated first. This initiates an extensor response in the fingers and the hand is maintained in the crawling position. A little air is then put into the anterior chamber for comfort and to give a good weightbearing base. Note that this splint is not used to stabilize the wrist. It is used to control fingers and thumb.

Use

1. To assist in early weightbearing exercise through a correctly positioned hand.
2. To assist hand position when crawling begins.
3. Used to control the thumb and fingers while graduated wrist extension against resistance is practised.

THE LEG GAITER

Method of application

This is a double chamber leg splint, which is applied with the zip fastener down the lateral side of the leg.

The patient should be standing comfortably with good arm positioning (splint controlled and weightbearing). The feet must be apart and turned straight forward. The upper edge of the splint should be up under the ischial tuberosity. The posterior chamber must be inflated first to a firm pressure. As it is inflated the patient's weight should be transferred over onto the weak foot. If this is done correctly and the foot is correctly positioned the inflation will bring the affected knee into mild flexion and the heel firmly down onto the floor. The patient will be bearing weight through the heel to a mildly flexed knee and a correctly positioned hip, thus inhibiting strong extensor antigravity thrust and a consequent build-up of spasticity.

Finally a little air is put into the anterior chamber to give comfort and to stabilize the knee. The patient is now comfortably stable and ready to practise transfer of weight over the affected side.

Use

1. For standing, with the therapist using her hands to give trunk pressures, to train trunk stability.
2. For gait training by stepping forwards, backwards and sideways with the sound leg.
3. For practice in weight transfers from side to side with both feet firmly on the ground.
4. For standing, practising with both knees bending and stretching, keeping the heels on the floor. This leads to standing on the affected leg alone and continuing with the affected knee bending and stretching.

Note: All the suggested exercises lead to a stable and strong knee and ankle. This gaiter is not intended as a splint for walking.

SUMMARY

These splints are seen as a vital aid in the rehabilitation of stroke patients and are used during therapy sessions.

They inhibit developing spasticity by controlling tonal patterns and allow a motor retraining programme to develop along the same lines as the motor development of the infant. They increase sensory input and give the stability necessary for early weightbearing.

The infant rolls before he crawls, crawls before he kneels, and kneels before he stands. This gives the developmental sequence which is copied in the advancing rehabilitation programme. On the other hand, some infants change the sequence to rolling to sitting to standing and this sequence is sometimes more useful for the elderly patient with a stiff lumbar spine and/or osteoarthritis of the knees.

This training includes the whole body, giving the hemiplegic arm a reasonable hope of recovery. Recovery begins with rotation of head, neck and trunk, leading on to regaining trunk stability and spreading to shoulder and hip recovery before progressing down each limb.

The patient must be taught and supervised in constant (day and night) positioning of his body in the spasticity-inhibiting patterns. It has to be remembered that the *aim* is to give back to the brain-damaged patient inhibitory control over abnormal patterns of movement, the *purpose* being to restore postural control. Successful inhibition of developing spasticity depends on adequate control of the distribution of muscle tone at all times while a planned and advancing motor development programme is undertaken. Restoration of the postural reflex mechanism with normal muscle tone is the ultimate aim.

ROLLING

The following points concerning training in rolling patterns are linked with the stages of motor development on p. 12:

1. Recovery begins with rotation of head, neck and trunk. Start rolling patterns by turning eyes and head in the direction of the roll. Where necessary the therapist attracts the patient's eyes in the direction of the roll and the roll follows the movement of the eyes and head.
2. Make use of the tonic labyrinthine and tonic neck reflexes. The position of the head has a fundamental bearing on muscle tone because of the receptors in the inner ear and in cervical joints.
3. Look at the patient's body as a whole and guard against any unwanted chain reaction which, with the brain damage of stroke and consequent imbalance of muscle tone, must not be allowed to follow antigravity patterns.

4. Successful rehabilitation depends on constant repetition of all therapeutic movements which work into inhibiting patterns.

5. Start with the trunk, but, at the same time, maintain inhibiting patterns in the limbs.

6. To recover postural stability and controlled movement, irradiation and the use of associated reactions to strengthen weak tone is invaluable, provided strong and adequate control of antigravity tone can be maintained.

7. Approximation, the compression of the trunk on an extremity, correctly applied, has much to contribute towards recovery. For example, compression through joints has the effect of encouraging extension, but much depends on the weightbearing base. Compression through the ball of the foot promotes an extensor thrust and this can have no place in the stroke programme. But, pressure under the heel stimulates dorsiflexion (see Fig. 26) and encourages knee flexion. Compression also stimulates joint proprioceptors.

Figures 33–41 represent just a few of the ways in which inhibitory control over antigravity tonal patterns may be maintained, while the progressive and advancing motor recovery programme is undertaken.

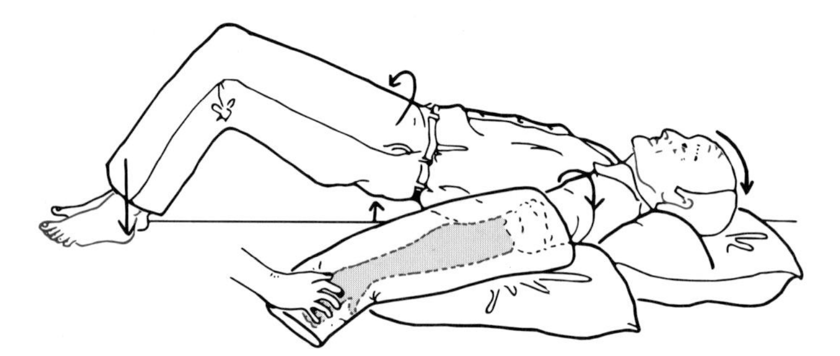

Fig. 33 The inflatable splint directs tonal flow into the extension pattern. Bridging, without the use of the long arm splint, increases the unwanted antigravity flexion pattern of the forearm.

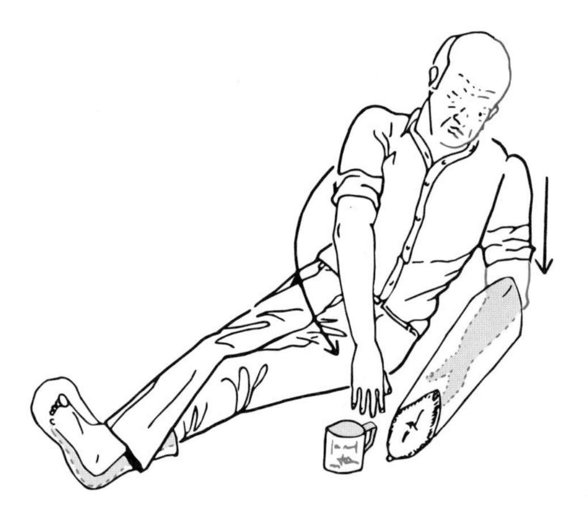

Fig. 34 Controlling tone in wrist and fingers with the half-arm splint. Early propping on the elbow, with outward rotation of the shoulder, increases shoulder stability.

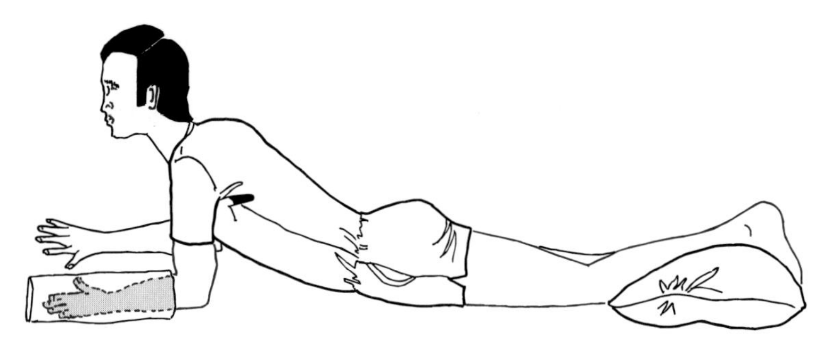

Fig. 35 Prone lying, propping on parallel forearms, working to gain stability of the outwardly rotated shoulder. The half-arm splint controls forearm position. The foot splint, with pressure through the heel, assists in inhibiting the unwanted extensor pattern, if it is brought into use here.

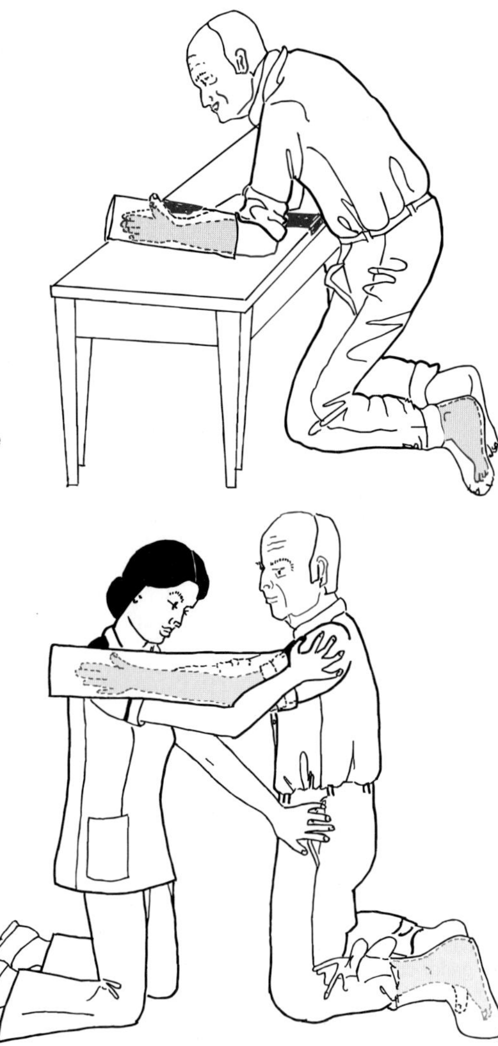

Fig. 36 Modified prone lying for the elderly. To be used when the lumbar spine is stiff and painful.

Fig. 37 Learning to transfer weight over to the affected side.

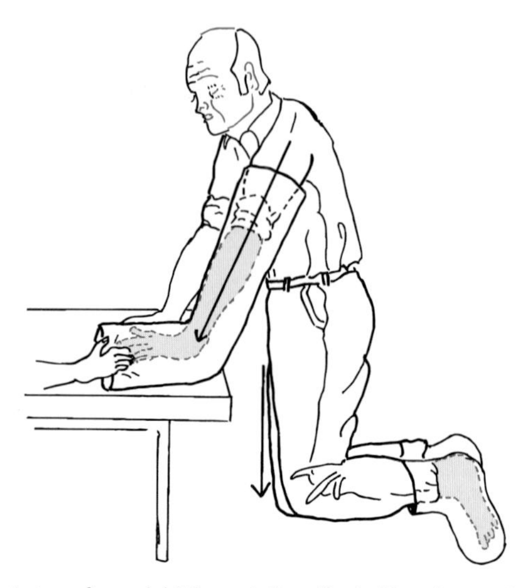

Fig. 38 Learning to transfer weight through the affected hand on an inhibited arm.

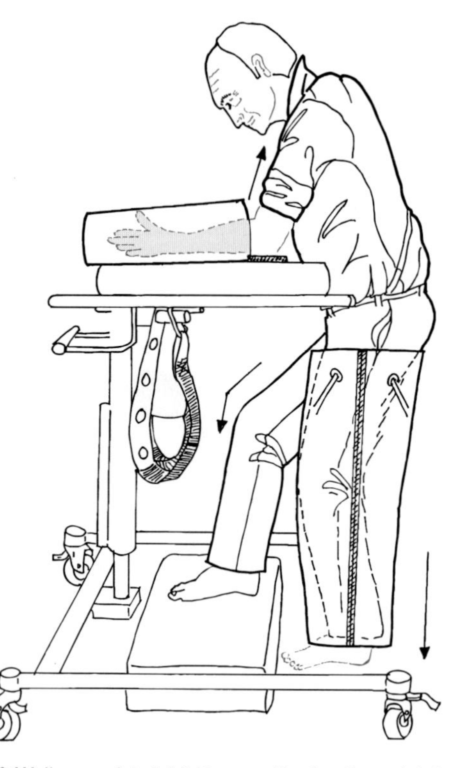

Fig. 39 The Arjo Lift Walker assists inhibiting positioning for weightbearing exercise. The leg gaiter controls the inhibiting leg pattern and the foot must not be moved. Only the sound foot steps up and down. Exercises will include standing on both feet and extending the head against resistance, bilateral knee bending, single knee bending while standing on the affected foot, training trunk stability, etc.

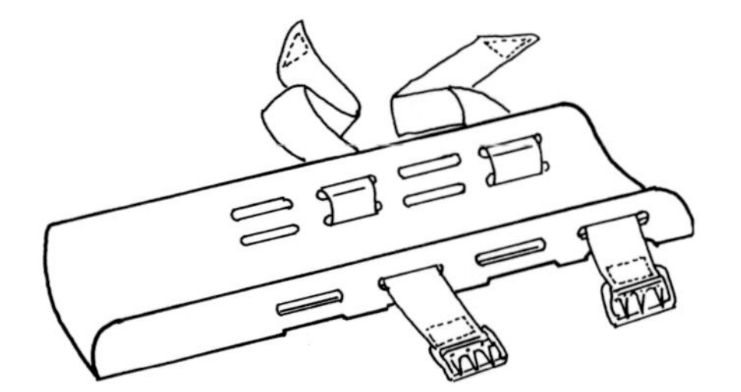

Fig. 40 A suggested gutter arm support, to be fixed to the arm of the chair.

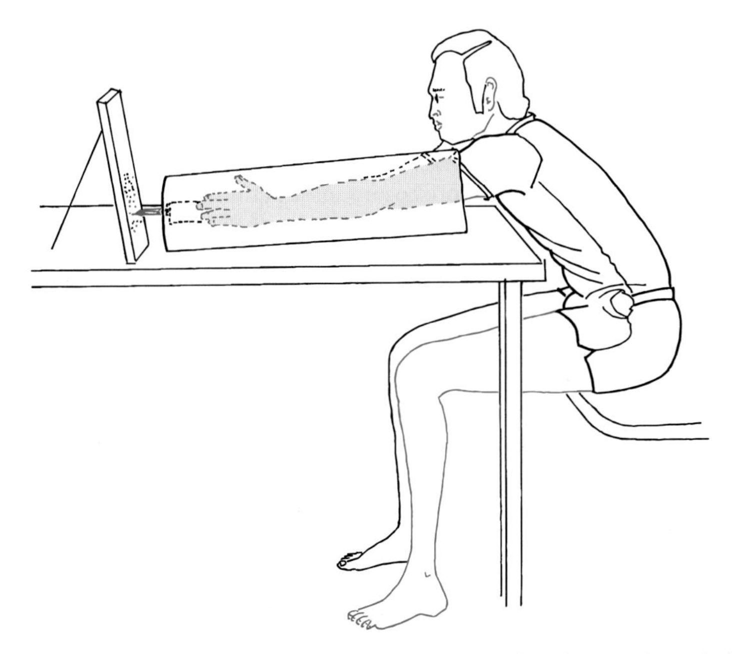

Fig. 41 With a pen fastened into the pressure splint, the patient draws a picture in dots. Shoulder protraction is used in reaching towards the drawing. Occupational therapy has much to offer to this positive recovery programme.

RESULTS WITH LONG-TERM PATIENTS

It became increasingly obvious as work in the long-term hospital went ahead that treatment results were greatly improved where pressure splints were integrated into the exercise routines. Clinical observation and comparison with former treatment results particularly seemed to demonstrate an often surprising recovery in arm function. However, there are always variables in any treatment approach; variables which must be considered and which make a true comparison of results impossible. Here, the patients' circumstances had changed. Where patients had sat around in wheelchairs for most of the day, with no standing balance and severe residual problems, particularly the problems associated with the hemiplegic arm, they still sat around in wheelchairs for much of the day, but a programme of careful arm positioning was undertaken and pressure splint control was used in exercise sessions.

To reverse the presenting problems associated with severe spasticity was, not unexpectedly, a slow, though not always impossible task, using a sensorimotor approach with pressure splints supplying stability with inhibitory positioning. Where extreme flaccidity was the problem, results were poor. With rehabilitation techniques that gave a positive boost to sensory input, some patients were able to respond and others were not. Sensorimotor integration depends on a continuous flow of sensory information. Somewhere, there had to be a need for even greater sensory input. Further consideration had to be given to sensory loss. All movements result from sensory stimulation by way of sight, hearing and touch. Movements are guided by sight and through the stimulation of the proprioceptors of muscles, tendons and joints which are activated by movement in the tissues. Sensory stimuli initiate and direct motor function. Proprioceptors are sensory nerve endings receptive to sensory stimuli. This was established elementary neurological understanding, a theme which, with further development, gave some missing answers (Johnstone 1976).

REFERENCES

Johnstone M 1976 The stroke patient: principles of rehabilitation. Churchill Livingstone, Edinburgh

5

SENSORY LOSS AND THE IMPORTANCE OF ASSESSMENT

ASSESSMENT OF SENSORY LOSS

Sensory loss may be a major barrier to successful rehabilitation and an early estimate of any disability in this area should be made. Postural sense, vision, sensation and abstract thought should be assessed as soon as possible.

There are four initial and very quick tests which may be used to indicate any sensory deficit in these areas. I have frequently found these tests most useful and I am grateful to Professor Bernard Isaacs (1987) who gave them to me with his free permission to use them. With a little practice none of these tests takes more than a minute. They give a very quick initial assessment of brain damage, usually associated with the nondominant lobe of the brain, and indicate the need to make a sound sensorimotor approach to rehabilitation.

1. Postural sense

Ask the patient to grasp the thumb of his affected hand with his sound hand. Repeat the task with the eyes covered but altering the position of the affected arm after the eyes are covered. The patient with defective proprioception will fail to find his thumb.

2. Vision

Hemianopia and visual agnosia must not be confused. (Agnosia is loss of the power to perceive.) Neglect of one half of space is very quickly demonstrated when two brightly coloured pens of contrasting colours are held in front of the patient, about 30 cm (12 inches) apart, and he fails to identify one of them.

Note: The patient with hemianopia will only see one pen but he will see both pens if they are interchanged in front of his eyes because he is able to follow the pen that moves into the blind half of his visual field. In cases of severe neglect of half of space, only one pen is seen even when they are moved so that they are in front of the patient and less than 2.5 cm (1 inch) apart. Even when they are interchanged in front of the patient's eyes he will not be able to follow the pen that moves into the blind half of his visual field.

3. Sensation

Cutaneous sensibility, or tactile sensation, ought to be tested. The patient is asked to identify a light touch on any part of the body without the help of the eyes. Two-point discrimination is also used to test deep pressure. The result of the test depends on the patient's ability to distinguish two points from one on the finger pulps, without using the eyes.

4. Abstract thought

Use a quick test, e.g. picture identification. The test suggested here will also uncover visual agnosia and neglect of the left half of space, and takes no more than a minute to carry out. A picture of a man and a woman is all that is needed, preferably a bride and groom, and the picture should be mounted for easy handling. The patient is shown the picture and asked a series of questions, beginning with 'What do you see?'.

If he cannot identify the picture he is asked:

- 'Is there a man in the picture?'
- 'Point to the man.'
- 'Is there anyone else?'
- 'Is there a woman?'
- 'Point to the woman.'
- 'What is the woman wearing?' . . . . . and so on.

Interpretation of the test is as follows:

a. Patients with visual agnosia fail completely.
b. Patients with neglect of the left half of space fail to identify the figure in the left half of the picture.
c. Patients with loss of abstract thought fail to give a general interpretation of the picture, for instance calling the bride 'a woman', or they misidentify the picture through misinterpreting a fundamental detail, for instance the bride may be described as a nurse.

Timing of assessment

Where sensorimotor disturbance is present, it is an established fact that, if the nondominant hemisphere is involved, the obstacles to rehabilitation may be severe. No two stroke patients present exactly the same problems. It is always necessary to carry out very careful and therefore accurate assessment of the damage resulting from the individual stroke.

It is also important to remember that performance will vary from day to day and, where severe damage is present, a reliable assessment for further prognosis cannot be made in the early days. Indeed, it will be a full month after onset before a prognosis assessment (with no sensory involvement) may be in any way reliable. Over many years, in my clinical studies, I have come to believe that all stroke patients have some degree of sensory loss, but I may have reached this conclusion because most of my time over a period of 30 years has been taken up with severely brain-damaged patients. Where sensory involvement is included, the time necessary to reach a reliable prognosis assessment will usually be at least 2 months. If parietal lobe syndrome is included, the prognosis assessment time will be 3–4 months. These figures depend on intensive treatment and correct handling.

DRAWING TESTS

These tests are frequently used to assist in making an accurate assessment, but they must be interpreted correctly. The drawings should be done using a separate sheet of paper for each drawing, with a felt-tipped pen, and using a firm clipboard to hold the paper in place.

Try to observe the patient's performance without his being aware that you are watching him.

Who should carry out these drawing tests? If there is an occupational therapist in the team, it is usually considered to be her job. The team must communicate with each other and make joint decisions and agree on practice, but only one therapist undertakes the drawing tests.

Interpretation

The following notes should be helpful:

1. Make allowances for left-handed drawings done by the right-handed patient.
2. Always note the position of the drawing on the page, remembering that patients with neglect of the left half of space place their drawings on the right half of the page.
3. Note the size of the drawing, remembering that demented patients tend to make very small drawings.
4. An elaborate detailed drawing tends to point to a high intellectual level prior to the stroke.
5. Note the placing of the parts of the body which may be disrupted, grossly misshapen, or missing in cases of agnosia.
6. Leaving out the left half of a drawing, for example a house, indicates visual agnosia, or severe neglect of the left half of space.
7. Incoherent drawing usually indicates receptive dysphasia or dyspraxia; repetitive scribbling should be noted as perseveration (tendency to experience difficulty in leaving one thought for another).
8. The drawing with a lateral lean, or the progressive lateral lean of repeated arrows drawn across a page, may indicate postural difficulties. A vertical arrow pointing upwards and not too small is drawn on the left side of the sheet of paper and the patient is asked to copy the arrow right across the page.

9. A clock drawn with numbers wandering outside the face indicates general brain damage, as distinct from the clock drawn with numbers omitted in cases of spatial neglect.

'Draw a man', 'Draw a house', and 'Draw a clock'

'Draw a man', 'Draw a house', and 'Draw a clock' are the tasks most frequently used in these tests. Copy drawings of these same subjects are very useful tests, particularly where agnosia, apraxia and spatial neglect on either side is suspected. Drawings to be copied ought to be done by the therapist in front of the patient. The drawing should then be moved upward so that it is immediately above the clean sheet of paper to be used by the patient and not alongside it.

Always stress that the ability to draw well does not matter. Always remember that each new drawing must be done on a fresh piece of paper and one drawing is completed before the next is attempted. Always sit quietly, a little behind the patient, while watching his performance; this should help him to relax and lose any embarrassment about the state of his drawing.

All therapists ought to be competent enough to undertake all tests and to understand their interpretation. Information about patient assessment, treatment, progress, etc must pass freely between team members, and they should be prepared to share their expertise, to cross each others' borders and truly integrate, to produce a satisfactory treatment programme which is in the best interests of the individual patient.

Examples of assessment drawings

Figures 42 and 43 are examples of assessment drawings from two patients. Both were the response to the request 'Draw a man'. The results of this test

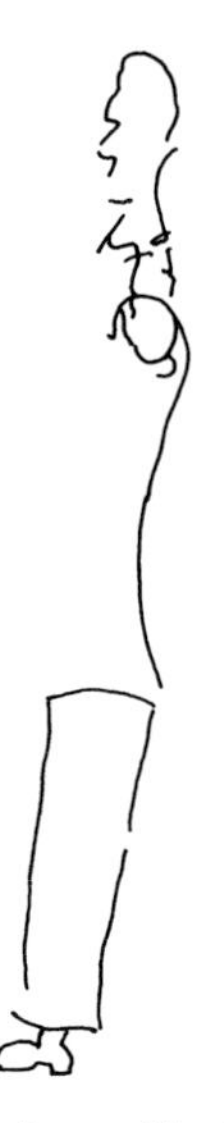

Fig. 42 Loss of body image. A drawing by a patient who had lost all sense of the position of his left arm in space. (60% of actual size.)

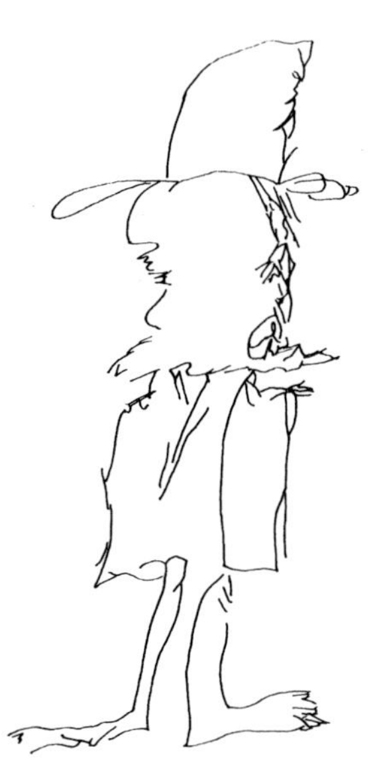

Fig. 43 Like Fig. 42, a drawing done in response to the request 'Draw a man'. Severe proprioceptive loss was isolated. (60% of actual size.)

are varied but the therapist who is well practised in presenting the test soon learns from experience how best to interpret the results. The initial drawing tests, which are presented as early as is practical after the onset of a stroke, can be a great help to the physiotherapist. Her concern is physical recovery, or the return of muscles and movement to normal function, and the quicker an overall picture is gained of the problems the patient is facing the better. The assistance and full cooperation of an experienced occupational therapist and a skilled speech therapist are of enormous help. Where relationships are right, each will share enough of her specialized skill to give common respect and understanding.

Figure 42 was drawn by a man who had lost all sense of the position of his left arm in space. Using the blindfold thumb finding test of postural sense described above, the patient failed to find his thumb. Next, still blindfolded, the position of his affected arm was altered and he was asked to copy the position of his affected arm with his sound arm. Again he failed, and each time the angle of the elbow joint was altered he continued to fail the test. This demonstrated marked loss of proprioceptive sense in the whole arm.

Figure 43, a rather bizarre drawing, was not quite so easy to interpret, but it also suggested a missing arm, this time the right arm. This was confusing until it was established that the patient was left-handed. The patient started with a large and positive attempt at drawing the head. After that the drawing became slow and she constantly returned to the head and added small uncertain strokes of the pen down the back of the head, a meaningless repetition of drawing on the already completed head. Her problem was perseveration, a tendency to experience difficulty in leaving one thought for the next when attempting a task. Further tests established proprioceptive loss in her right arm.

Both patients had serious problems which had to be faced. The use of the pressure splint and pressure techniques had given a valuable boost to sensory input, but the question still remained, why were some patients able to respond while others were not? These two were among those who did not respond; that is, they did not respond until one more technique was added to the recovery programme.

NEGLECT

This condition occurs in nondominant paralysis. It may be classified into five types.

1. A condition in which the patient is not aware of anything over the midline. This includes half of his body and, as far as he is concerned, nothing exists in that half of space. Figure 42 does not demonstrate neglect. Had it done so, the drawing would have been placed towards the right side of the paper.
2. Loss of body image. The patient will take the tester's hand only if it is placed on his sound side ('hand test').
3. The extra limb. The patient will refer to an extra limb by name, e.g. 'My little friend George'. The perceived extra limb will suddenly disappear, but the patient will believe it had been there; or, 'finding an extra limb' in bed beside him may cause him great embarrassment.
4. Anosognosia (see below), or denial of disability. For example, a severely disabled patient is asked 'Can you ride a bicycle?' and he replies that he can.
5. Defects in personality. The patient may appear garrulous, superficial or shallow, or may exhibit a shallow sense of humour. High pressure speech may be a feature. The therapist must work at establishing a good relationship with the patient.

Tests for neglect

The two pen test and copying a drawing may be used to uncover problems of neglect. The thumb finding test is not valid where neglect is present.

Anosognosia

This is the failure to recognize the disability involving the forgotten half of the body, i.e. neglect or denial of ownership of the affected limbs. When neglect is complicated by dense anosognosia with both visual and sensory problems, the rehabilitation team is faced with probably the most difficult of all handicaps to be overcome. Nevertheless, even patients with this disability should not be simply regarded as having poor prospects for recovery of independence, provided there is not an underlying and serious medical condition. As we begin to understand more about the problems presenting with such a patient, we begin to see there may be a way ahead.

This indicates the importance of making a reliable assessment, and for therapists and doctors to understand the problems which treatment must address. Rehabilitation will range from a relatively uncomplicated recovery of lost physical ability to facing these new very difficult barriers where severe neglect has become the problem.

A patient with anosognosia

Figures 44–46 show the assessment drawings done by a patient who presented with severe problems. She was admitted to the long-term hospital 4 weeks after the onset of a stroke. Her admission request stated that she was not expected to recover sufficiently to go home. Nevertheless she was given a bed in the specialized stroke unit to give her the proverbial dog's chance. She was to stay in this unit for 1 month before a decision about her future would be made.

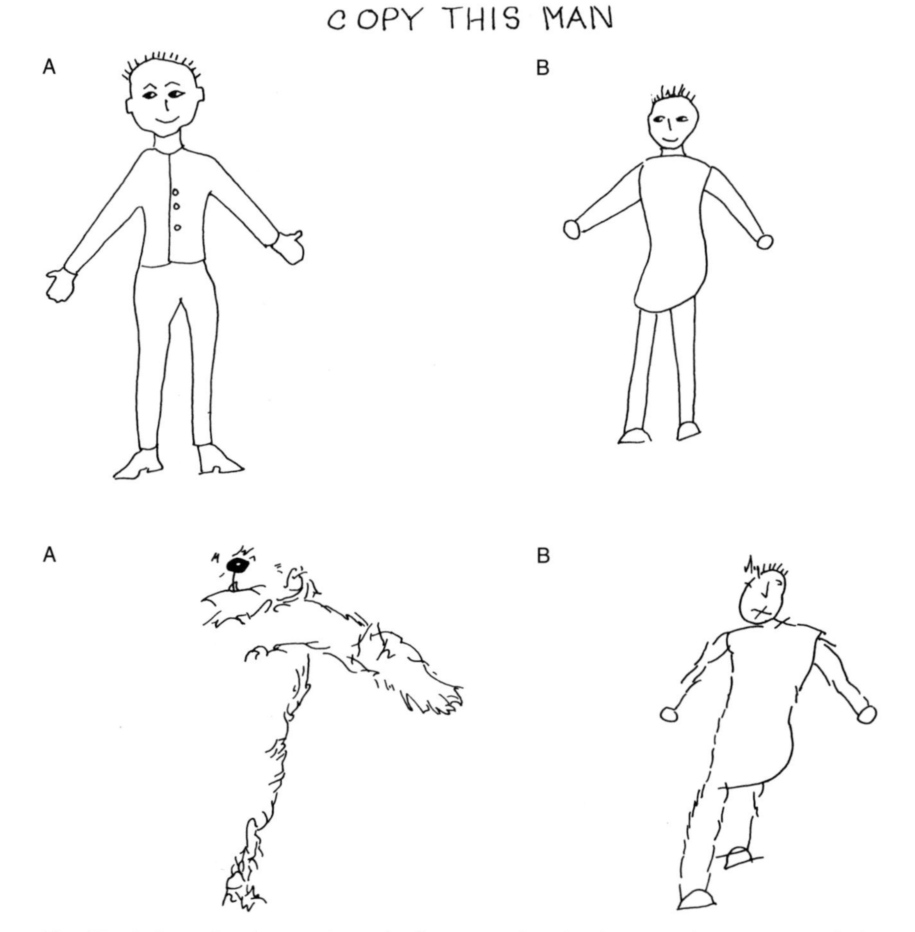

Fig. 44 A. Copy drawing test 1 month after onset of stroke. Interpretation: severe neglect; the patient was not aware of anything across the midline. B. The same test repeated 1 month later. All possible pressure techniques with intensive physiotherapy had been used. Interpretation: positive recovery was going well. It was decided to continue with this regime. (30% of actual size.)

COPY THIS CLOCK

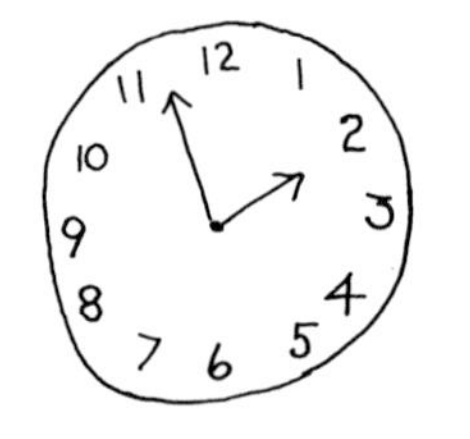

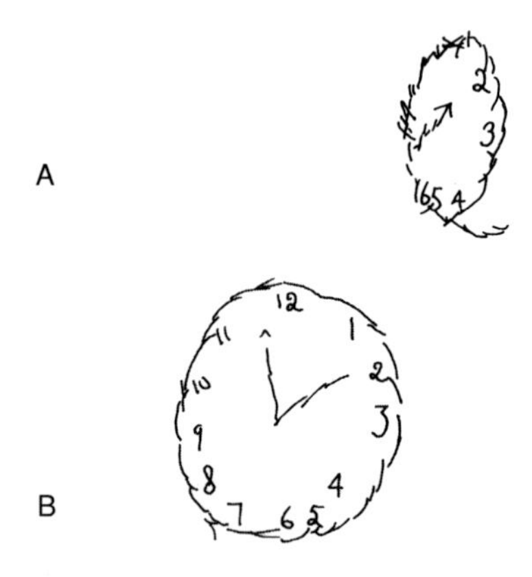

Fig. 45 A and B. Test drawings done by the same patient at the same times as those in Fig. 44 A and B. Each drawing was done on a separate piece of paper. (30% of actual size.)

This patient had no secure sitting balance and she sprawled backwards with her legs stretched out in extension. The position of her head gave an instant clue to the nature of her disability; it dropped backwards, supported by the high back of the chair and at all times rotated away from her disabled side. Any approach made on her disabled side was ignored. One day after admission to the long-term hospital she was propped up into an acceptable sitting position and presented with drawing tests.

Further tests revealed dense anosognosia: the patient failed to identify her own clothing; visual agnosia was marked; she failed to recognize any part of her own body on her affected side; nothing existed for her over the midline, and yet she wrapped her affected arm in a shawl and cuddled it, calling it her ‘wee papoose’. Placing her, both in and out of bed, so that she was approached at all times on her affected side, in an attempt to increase sensory stimulation, with all stimuli bombarding her affected side, and increased by pressure from the inflatable splints, led to a marked response.

One month later she was presented with the same drawing tests. She did not appear to have made much progress and she still turned her head to

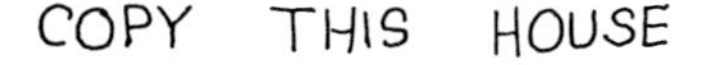

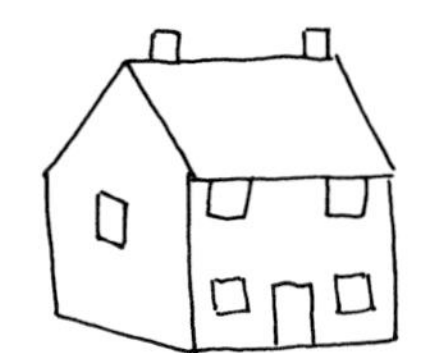

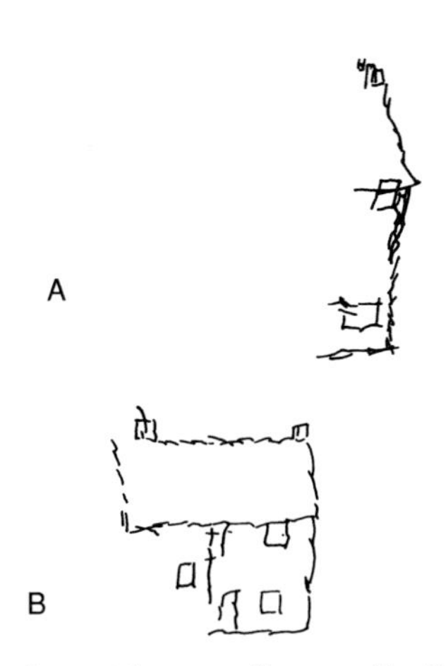

Fig. 46 A and B. The third test done at the same times and by the same patient as Figs 44 and 45. (30% of actual size.) Figs 44–46 are classic drawings demonstrating severe neglect, with advancing and very hopeful signs of recovery.

the sound side. The clinical meeting where her future would be decided took place the next day. The decision that she should be sent back to the long-term ward for permanent care was almost unanimous, until the team members were presented with the results of her drawing tests. She continued to rehabilitate in the stroke unit.

Formerly, in severe cases of this nature, rehabilitation had failed, but now an 'intermittent pressure' technique (see below) had been added to the treatment regime, and seemed to present an answer to loss of proprioceptive sense.

A NEED FOR ALTERING PRESSURES?

Physical rehabilitation had met with success where primitive reflex movement, present at birth, had been taken as the basis (using inhibiting patterns) on which to rebuild a recovery programme, but this had failed where there was severe sensory loss. Why not go even further back in development, when considering sensory loss, and consider sensory development in the fetus. The newborn infant arrives with an inbuilt sensory system, programmed into fetal development from about the third to the ninth month by pressure and altering pressures. All the time the fetus grows he is enclosed in a bag of fluid where pressures continually alter as the mother moves, breathes and goes about her daily duties. The fetus is subjected to sensory input from touch, movement and altering pressures. Where exercises were undertaken while a limb was enclosed in an inflatable splint, pressures altered, but was this enough? The pressure splint supplied touch, and all over even pressure, but it seemed to be deficient in the need to stimulate proprioceptors by the addition of adequate altering pressures.

A CLINICAL TRIAL OF THE INFLATABLE PRESSURE SPLINT

Physiotherapists were sceptical. They wanted scientific proof that inflatable pressure splints had any useful part to play in physical recovery of the stroke patient. However, as an invited speaker, presenting a paper on muscle tone and the stroke patient, I found myself sharing a lecture platform with Dr E G Walsh of the Department of Physiology at the medical school of Edinburgh University. He and his research team, using apparatus designed and built in Edinburgh by Dr Walsh, were working on measurements of muscle tone using printed motors as torque generators (Walsh et al 1980). (Among other things I picked up an excellent definition: 'Resting muscle tone is defined as the resistance offered by relaxed muscle to passive stretch. It is comparable to the restoring force exerted by a spring in response to extension.')

After the meeting Dr Walsh offered to set up a trial which, he believed, would give me the evidence I needed to support the claims I made for the use of pressure splints in stroke care. He asked me to produce a number of patients presenting with severe arm spasticity after stroke. At that time, from among the patients in a long-term hospital, this was not difficult to do. I chose nine patients and examined them very carefully. Out of the nine I decided one was not suitable for the trial. She was an elderly lady with a severe emotional and anxiety state amounting to paranoia and, in such a case, experience has taught me that no amount of treatment is effective unless the adverse emotional state (a considerable contributing factor in the build-up of spasticity) can be dealt with. In her case this had not been possible; as fast as one worry was dealt with and removed, the next worry moved in and became an obsession. To the present day I still find it very difficult to deal with such an extreme case. Eight patients were tested.

TEST OF WRIST SPASTICITY

For the purpose of our study we decided to test wrist spasticity. All eight patients were tested in the position of greatest flexor spasticity, that is, sitting with flexed elbow, wrist and fingers, with head and neck rotated and flexed towards the affected hand, thus allowing asymmetrical tonic neck flexion to act against us by increasing tone in the wrist flexors. With each patient seated in this position we tested wrist spasticity (wrist compliance measurement) using the Walsh machine. The man-to-machine link was a printed motor, invented in France in the early 1950s. Forces were applied to the limb resulting in flexion and extension of the wrist and the resulting mechanical displacement was analysed. An EMG was recorded from flexor and extensor muscles.

Immediately after this control test an orally inflated pressure splint was applied to the arm, with the arm in the full inhibiting pattern of extension of the elbow, wrist and fingers and extension with abduction of the thumb. In the sitting position the splinted arm was given pillow support with the shoulder in outward rotation. The treatment span I had recommended during the previous 2 years as a suitable time to produce a reduction in spasticity had been 1 hour, but after consultation we decided to set the clock timer for 70 minutes. At the end of the agreed time, the splint was removed and the wrist again tested with the patient back in the original position of maximum spasticity build-up. All eight patients were tested in this way and all showed a reduction in wrist spasticity at the end of the test. The printout in Figure 47 shows our best result. We had tested seven patients with major arm spasticity who were 3–5 months post-stroke and an eighth patient with severe spasticity who was 2 years post-stroke.

INTERPRETATION OF THE TEST

Figure 47 illustrates the test result on patient number eight.

Mrs E L had spasticity of the left wrist. The control trace showed a stiff response, with clonic oscillations following applications of extensor force. The phasic EMG spikes seen in flexors are related to clonic oscillations. There was a high level of resting tonic flexor EMG.

After use of the pressure splint, the clonic activity had more or less gone, with just one slight oscillation during extension. Associated with this, the tonic and phasic flexor EMG was much reduced. The response became much more 'plastic' with moulding of the wrist into extension as the flexors yielded.

I had not expected that we would record anything approaching a 'good' result as the tests were deliberately carried out with all patients sitting in the position of maximum flexor spasticity of the arm. I feel confident that we tested a sufficient number of cases to be able to state that the orally inflated pressure splint, carefully applied to hold the arm in the reflex inhibiting position, reduces unwanted spasticity and therefore becomes a useful tool in the hands of expert therapists (both physiotherapists and occupational therapists) and nurses. If nurses are not taught to use inhibiting patterns and the need to apply the full arm splint for some of the handling techniques, much valuable rehabilitation time is lost.

As far as I know the carry-over effect of this treatment has not been established. However, the task for therapists is to capitalize on the improved climate for rehabilitation, using the techniques suggested here in a realistic and feasible way, and greatly improving treatment results.

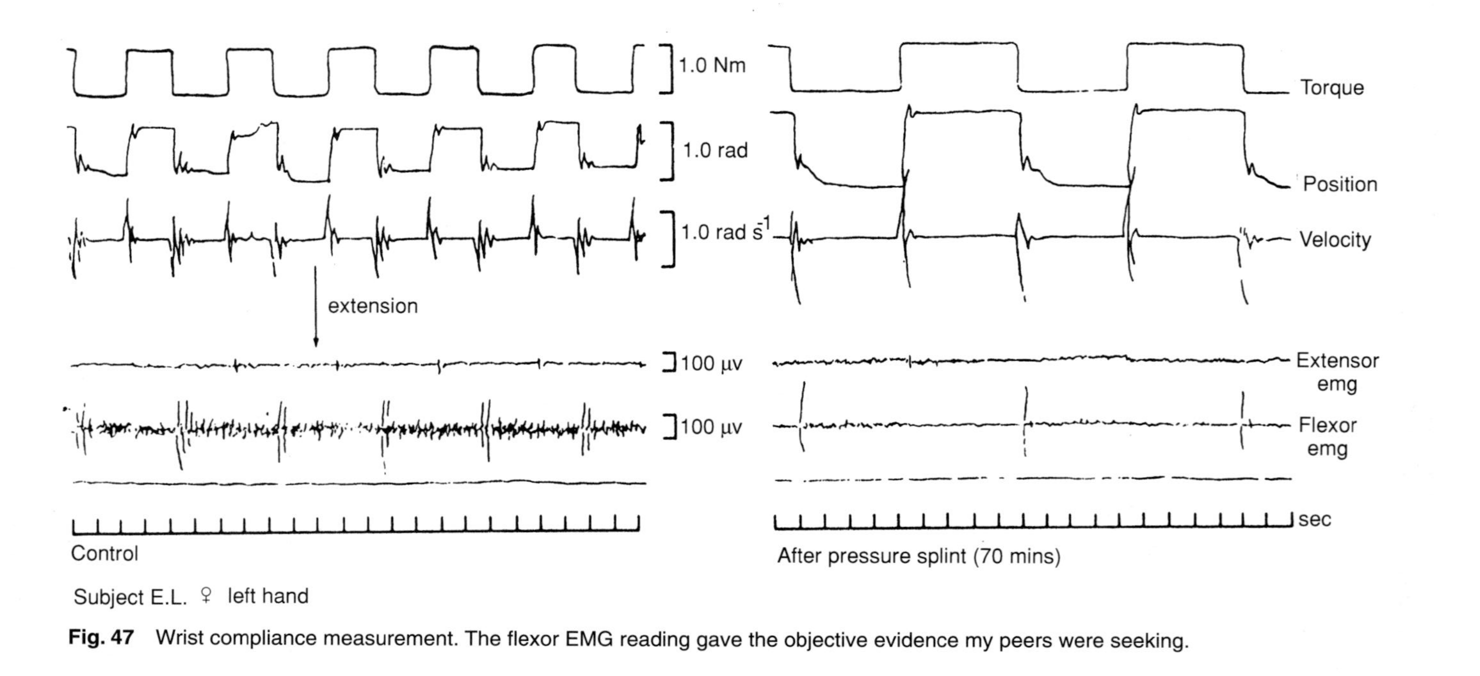

Fig. 47 Wrist compliance measurement. The flexor EMG reading gave the objective evidence my peers were seeking.

CONCLUSIONS FROM THE STUDY

We concluded that, as treatment for the hemiplegic arm is based on the careful use of reflex inhibition and an attempt to facilitate by working into inhibitory patterns, the physiotherapy profession cannot afford to ignore the valuable contribution to treatment offered by the skilled use of the orally inflatable sustained pressure splint.

THE INTERMITTENT PRESSURE TECHNIQUE

SEVERE PROPRIOCEPTIVE LOSS IN THE HEMIPLEGIC ARM

Continuing to meet with failure in recovery of the hemiplegic arm where severe proprioceptive loss was found, it seemed there had to be some way of stepping up sensory input with alternating pressures until the necessary response was gained. Sustained pressure splint support had made it possible to bear weight through the arm and bombard joint proprioceptors, but something had to be done to further stimulate muscle proprioceptors. The following quotation from George Adam's book (1974), *Cerebrovascular Disability and the Ageing Brain*, had had a profound effect on my thinking:

> *Defective proprioception denies the patient the assured knowledge of joint position and movement essential to the recovery of mobility. The servo system concerned in antigravity and postural mechanisms is dependent on it, and even when motor power and intellect are well preserved, loss of proprioception results in severe and persistent handicap.*

This presented a challenge; there had to be an answer.

Returning to the area of sensory development before birth and the altering pressures exerted on the fetus, the mother's breathing sequence supplies constant and regular altering pressures; clearly it seemed there was a vital need to add an intermittent pressure technique to the recovery programme. This would attempt to mimic the mother's breathing pattern and bombard muscle proprioceptors, giving movement within the tissues. It would also take care of the fact that sensory nerves accommodate sustained pressure.

Again, in the long-term hospital, finding patients with proprioceptive loss was not a problem. Four patients who had already failed to rehabilitate over several weeks in the specialized stroke unit and who had presented with severe proprioceptive loss continued in the unit with the same routine, but intermittent pressure was added to their daily treatment programme. At first any improvement in clinical results was not apparent but, over a period of 4–8 weeks, all recovered useful motor control. I have continued this regime ever since and I have no hesitation in stating that where there is loss of proprioceptive sense, it is essential to add intermittent pressure to the rehabilitation programme.

The test drawings shown in Figures 44–46 were all done by the patient who has been described earlier in this chapter. She came into our stroke unit

4 weeks after the onset of a severe stroke and 1 year after we had started using intermittent pressure. Her initial assessment results meant that she was at once a candidate for intermittent pressure. The clinical results were very exciting. Where before there had been failure in arm recovery, now there was success. However, success was not always so rapid. During the next 4 years in the same specialized stroke unit, admitting a number of patients who had not had strokes very recently, the results were less exciting. For example, one patient had 2 years of intermittent pressure before there was a breakthrough into sensory recovery. The results suggested that treatment should begin as soon as possible after the onset of a stroke, but this has long been a rule that should be followed in all treatment.

CONTRAINDICATIONS

This type of mechanical alteration in pressure should not be used on patients in acute pulmonary oedema. It should be used with caution on those with congestive heart failure or where pre-existing deep vein thrombosis is suspected. Where it has been thought necessary to prescribe an anticoagulant, once the prothrombin rate has been stabilized, intermittent pressure may be used. If in doubt consult the physician.

CAUTION

Intermittent pressure should not be used as a technique to reduce spasticity. The use of very high pressure results in hypoxia. It has been shown by other workers that 25 minutes of hypoxia can alter sensation of the four modalities, touch and pressure disappearing before temperature and pain. Immediately after treatment using very high pressure the limb may appear to show marked reduction in spasticity because of hypoxia, but, if the treatment is continued, excessive spasticity will be the end result. Besides, very high pressures interfering with blood flow are clearly contraindicated in all stroke treatment.

MECHANICAL PRESSURE PUMPS

There are various pumps on the market. The treatment suggested here was undertaken with the introduction of the British Flowpulse 1100 machine, supplied by Huntleigh Medical Ltd. This machine offered:

— pressure: variable, 20–100 mmHg
— inflation time: variable, in steps 3 seconds – 4 minutes
— deflation time: variable, in steps 3 seconds – 4 minutes
— treatment time: variable, up to 1 hour.

Where it was necessary to include intermittent pressure in the treatment programme because of gross loss of proprioceptive sense, I gave a twice-daily session of intermittent treatment with the Flowpulse machine. Each session lasted for 45 minutes; this time was arbitrary, and not based on reasoned or clinical examination. It was set simply by the amount of hours available in a busy working day.

After a careful research study on blood flows, involving Dr Joan Gelman of the Edinburgh University Physiology Department, we reached the conclusion that this machine should only be used on the hemiplegic limb provided meticulously correct pressures are employed.

In *Restoration of Motor Function in the Stroke Patient* (Johnstone 1983, 1987) I published our findings as follows:

> We offer here a clear indication of the pressures to be used:
> P1, 40 mmHg 3 seconds.
> P2, 10 mmHg 3 seconds. Time, 45 minutes.

To date, the sleeves supplied with intermittent pressure machines are not transparent, making it difficult to establish that the patient's arm and hand are fully maintained in the inhibitory pattern. I use the URIAS see-through splint. (For information on available sources of supply see Appendix.) I inflate this splint by mouth. This warms the inner plastic sheath so that it moulds to the limb and makes sure that all over even pressure is offered to the limb. This will not cause harmful constriction and assists in maintaining the recovery arm and hand position. When fully inflated by mouth (pressure must not exceed 40 mmHg) it is clipped off, attached to the machine, and the machine is then switched on. As soon as the pressure gauge is registering the required pressure cycle, the clip is opened on the splint.

Sometimes neglect persists in the patient's foot. In this case a pressure boot supplied with the machine is used and pressures alternate between arm and leg. When applying the boot make sure the patient's heel is right back into the heel of the boot. Pressure must be applied through the heel and not through the front of the foot (see Fig. 26). The treatment is applied with the patient sitting, correctly positioned in a suitable chair with support for the splinted arm. If the longer full leg sleeve is used to take in the knee, special care must be taken in lying, to maintain the hip in inward rotation with the leg in slight elevation.

Some of the pressure machines presently on the market do not have a deflation time. In this situation, the deflation time will be the resting period between inflation and deflation as the intermittent cycle takes place.

CONCLUSION

Where severe handicap is present because the servo system concerned in antigravity and postural mechanisms lacks proprioception, the pressure splint may be used to supply the necessary stimulation to bridge the gap. The sensorimotor approach to stroke rehabilitation as described here is a reasoned and satisfying approach which gives consistently good results. With a breakdown in the finely balanced facilitatory–inhibitory principle on which the neuromuscular system depends, therapists and all who care for stroke patients must act as an extended facilitatory–inhibitory agent until normal responses are re-established and cortical control regained. This means that all should understand the inhibiting positions and be able to apply the splints correctly, and in particular, the arm splint.

If we fail in this basic need is it the fault of the physiotherapist? Is it a failure to communicate with families? Are physiotherapists in the right place or should there be more of them in the home and fewer of them in hospitals? Are there enough to go round? These are questions that still need to be answered.

It is necessary to work out a pressure splint procedure, or specialized techniques, that will assist the development of the splint as an effective tool to stabilize limbs. At the same time, a build-up of unwanted antigravity tone must be inhibited while an advancing rehabilitation programme based on neuromotor development is implemented.

It should also be remembered that the Golgi tendon organs, the proprioceptors in the musculotendinous junctions, have an inhibitory influence on the motoneurone pools of their own muscles when stretch is applied.

All these facts would seem to substantiate the belief that there is a quite vital need to add inflatable splint techniques to any realistic approach to rehabilitation of the stroke patient.

REFERENCES

Adams G F 1974 Cerebrovascular disability and the ageing brain. Churchill Livingstone, Edinburgh

Johnstone M 1983, 1987 Restoration of motor function in the stroke patient, 2nd and 3rd edns. Churchill Livingstone, Edinburgh

Isaacs B 1971 Identification of disability in the stroke patient. Modern Geriatrics 1: 6

Walsh E G, Lakie M, Wright G W, Tsementzis S A 1980 Measurements of muscle tone using printed motors as torque generators. MEP 9: 3

6

GENERAL ASSESSMENT AND PROBLEM SOLVING

GENERAL ASSESSMENT

It is important to remember that each patient's needs will be established by accurate assessment. Very careful assessment is necessary so that the particular problems of each patient may be diagnosed, understood, and approached in a positive way. As already shown, the problems may include motor loss and/or sensory loss, and the consequent problems of sensorimotor function and perceptual difficulties. However, there are other difficulties. These may concern intellectual function, communication, family or employment, or be of a psychological or social nature. It is a daunting list, but this only makes it all the more urgently necessary to uncover the difficulties that may stand in the way of recovery and a return to normal living. It has to be remembered, for example, that a breakdown in a marriage relationship that has led to many years of unhappy acceptance of an unsatisfactory way of life can, after the onset of a stroke, completely block the necessary hopeful approach to rehabilitation that must be made by the patient himself, with family back-up if success is to be achieved. Assessment must include the home background.

ASSESSMENT OF MUSCLE TONE

The first priority of the physiotherapist in the clinical field is to understand the normal and the disruption of the normal that occurs in the stroke patient with the loss of postural control, and then to go straight to the heart of the matter by making an accurate assessment of the patient's state of muscle tone. Reliable assessment of the state of muscle tone is not a skill that can be taught in the classroom. It is an ability that can only be taught and developed in the clinical setting, with a hands-on approach, until the student is able to use techniques to divert, shift and therapeutically use tonal patterns to meet the needs of the individual patient. The physiotherapist feels the patient's tonal distribution, examining the patterns when she stimulates extra tonal input by bringing in head movements, or when she promotes overflow of tone which is stimulated by movements of the sound half of the body. (Such a simple action as yawning will frequently be seen to step up unwanted flexor tone in the forearm.)

A quick and provisional assessment of the patient's tonal state may be made by moving a disabled limb into the total inhibiting pattern. Where spasticity (or hypertonicity) is present, the further the limb is passively moved by the therapist into the inhibitory pattern, the more resistant it becomes. Unaided, the limb will drift at all times into the total pattern of spasticity and will be resistant to movement into the inhibiting pattern when handled by another person. On the other hand, where the limb gives no resistance but is heavy to handle (the 'floppy doll' limb) flaccidity (or hypotonicity) is present. The patient will have lost his placing response, he will be unable to support the limb against gravity and it will feel heavy and abnormally relaxed if handled by another person.

In stroke rehabilitation it is important to remember that immediately post-stroke there is no spasticity but that spasticity will develop very rapidly in many cases if measures are not taken to prevent it. Even the flaccid limb will eventually show signs of developing spasticity, which is usually first noted in the fingers. Therefore it is important to use careful positioning in inhibitory patterns from the early days and to practise the special pressure techniques necessary to divert tone into the inhibiting patterns and to increase tone in these patterns.

A more detailed and accurate assessment will be made in the following way. With the patient lying in the supine position, the lower half of his body is carefully placed and supported with pillows in a relaxed inhibitory pattern, while the arm is tested. Grading may be represented by scores of 1–5: 5 representing normal tone with no associated reactions. Six tests to grade the state of muscle tone may be carried out.

1. Can the patient hold his arm in elevation (vertical), it having been placed there?
2. Can he lower the extended arm through abduction from elevation to horizontal?

3. Can he return the arm to position 1?
4. With his arm in elevation, can he bend his elbow to touch the top of his head with his forearm in supination?
5. Can he return the arm to position 4, staying in supination?
6. Can he extend the arm in elevation with outward rotation while he carries out a grasp and release exercise with his hand?

It will be noted that tests 1–5 are progressively more difficult. Test 6 represents the normal.

To give an example, when undertaking test number 1 the therapist will place the patient's arm in elevation (without considering joint rotation) simply to find out if he is able to maintain this placed position. In many cases in the early days of treatment the patient cannot maintain even this fairly simple position, regardless of the shoulder pattern. At once the therapist understands the need to apply the long arm splint in the fully inhibiting pattern for the elbow, wrist and fingers, giving the arm the necessary stability while work on the trunk is undertaken.

Primarily, it is the business of rehabilitation therapists (and this includes rehabilitation nurses) to begin taking measures to deal with the effects of abnormal muscle tone as soon as possible after the onset of a stroke. For example, it is much better to make an early attempt to control developing spasticity than to attempt later to reverse the patterns of severe spasticity which have so often developed weeks or months after the onset of a stroke.

OTHER PROBLEMS

If the hoped for physical recovery of muscles and movement is to become a reality, it should not be surprising that restoration of normal muscle tone is considered here to be a first priority in rehabilitation with much of this book devoted to the need to restore postural control. However, there are other problems and the business of assessment is to uncover these problems so that each patient will have a tailor-made rehabilitation programme, which caters for his individual needs and is built into his physical programme.

To summarize the ground so far covered, these problems may include any of the following:

1. Loss of proprioceptive sense which leads to disturbance of body image, body image being the ability to feel a limb, to appreciate the movements of the joints and to appreciate the limb's place in space and its relationship to the body. Many patients have difficulties which present as agnosia (difficulty in recognition) and this may go as far as neglect or denial of ownership (anosognosia), or may even include denial of paralysis. Proprioceptive sense automatically controls antigravity and postural mechanisms and, without this control, the resulting severe handicap poses an enormous problem, the stability of sustained posture being essential for purposeful movement.

2. Impairment of tactile sensation with impairment of the ability to recognize objects by their shape, size and texture when held in the hand with the eyes shut (tactile agnosia, astereognosis), and impairment of coordination of

sensory input which gives disturbance of spatial relationships. If the brain is no longer aware of body image the patient will be incapable of determining his position in space. (Sensory messages from the proprioceptors of muscles and joints, from the proprioceptors of the neck in response to movement of the head, and changes in muscle tone by stimulation of the labyrinths all contribute to the brain's awareness of body image.)

3. Apraxic problems which result from a disturbance of visuospatial orientation. Because of the disorder of body image, these lead to an inability to deal effectively with or manipulate objects, e.g. dressing apraxia.

4. Problems in carrying out voluntary actions using objects in the environment (or space), or inability to copy designs of more than one dimension, usually recognized as constructional apraxia (e.g. 'Copy a box').

5. Problems of left–right discrimination.

6. Disturbances in visual perception which may include the inability to distinguish between vertical and horizontal positioning of an object held up in space. This is visual agnosia which must be recognized as a perceptual difficulty and not as blindness. The patient can see the object but he cannot assess its position in relationship to his own body image. If visual agnosia is present as the result of a bilateral lesion the effect is devastating. Where lesions are unilateral, compensation may be made. The patient who keeps bumping into objects and misjudging distances ought to be tested for visual agnosia. (Hemianopia is a quite different condition and does concern blindness of half of the visual field.)

Apraxic problems

These problems are often found to be present where there is no severe paralysis, and they fall into two types.

1. *Ideomotor apraxia.* The patient is incapable of carrying out purposeful movement on command, or of imitating unaccustomed gestures, while routine, automatic gestures and activities will still be performed. For example, if brushing his teeth was a former routine action and he is presented with his toothbrush he will brush his teeth because the action is automatic. However, if he is told to polish a horse brass with the toothbrush he will fail to carry out this new idea which is not automatic.

2. *Ideational apraxia.* The patient will fail in the automatic task. He will not brush his teeth when presented with his toothbrush. (Study of the Greek derivations can help our understanding. For example, there is a word 'ideopraxist', one who is impelled to carry out an idea, from the Greek *idea*, 'idea' and *praxis*, 'doing'.)

An understanding of these problems is essential if an intelligent approach is to be made to rehabilitation. With understanding, ideomotor disability may often be turned into successful movement. The patient may fail completely if he is given supporting assistance in standing and asked to concentrate on his leg movement and walk. However, if a cup of coffee is placed on a table on the other side of the room and he is told: 'There is your coffee. Go and get it', he will step out and cross the room.

One of the essential exercises in treating this kind of disability is the floor exercise where the patient clasps his hands, holding them up above his head, and rolls over and over across the full length of the room. Having mastered this he is taught to repeat it over and over again for as long as his exercise tolerance will allow.

Problems resulting from damage to the dominant and nondominant lobes

Where sensory loss is at a high functional level, the many difficulties which may be included in the parietal lobe syndrome are involved, and the problems presented may often seem insoluble. Some of these problems have already been introduced in Chapter 5 and now, under general assessment, more are needed. To avoid confusion and to help clarify the problems assessment may uncover, it can be useful to consider separately the dominant and nondominant lobes of the brain.

The dominant lobe is usually the left brain with a right-handed patient, but this is not always so. First find which is the patient's preferred hand. Family help may be needed to establish this.

The dominant lobe is concerned with logical, mathematical and communicating functions. Any of the following disabilities may be present:

1. Logic may be missing, and the unfortunate patient is labelled as one who does not try.
2. Disorders of speech.
3. Reading difficulty.
4. Writing difficulty (dysgraphia).
5. Arithmetic difficulty: simple mental arithmetic and adding (dyscalculia).
6. Bilateral apraxia; ideomotor, as already described.
7. Tactile astereognosis, as already described.
8. Postural difficulties, which may show as a lateral lean. (See also the 'pusher syndrome').
9. Right–left disorientation: difficulty in identifying right and left.
10. Finger agnosia: the patient has difficulty in identifying his fingers.

Remember to make allowances for any difficulty which already existed before the stroke. Again family help may be needed.

The nondominant lobe, usually the right brain, is the 'picture' brain, which interprets what is happening to the body or the environment. Any of the following disabilities may be present:

1. Disturbance of body image.
2. Neglect or denial of ownership of the affected limbs (anosognosia).
3. Disorder of spatial judgment.
4. Visual agnosia: a perceptual disturbance giving difficulty in recognition or failure to interpret what is seen.
5. Postural difficulties.
6. Constructional apraxia.
7. Tactile astereognosis.

These are formidable lists but all these disabilities will not present in any one patient. It is usually (but not always) less difficult to deal with dominant lobe damage than with nondominant damage. It is necessary to uncover any difficulties and, where necessary, to make allowances and to offer extra help. Obviously where there is parietal lobe involvement, or where the latter must be excluded, careful assessment must be undertaken, and this is where the skilled occupational therapist has much to offer. However, she may not always be available and, in any case, the physiotherapist ought to be able to carry out the basic tests that will help in her programme planning.

Using these lists of possible disabilities and becoming well practised in the basic tests presented to assess sensory loss, it will be found that it is possible to build up a fairly accurate picture of the problems the individual patient has to face. Over many years of clinical experience, setting out to restore normal movement, I found that an exercise programme based on neuromotor development gave a significant and positive boost to making good the sensory loss.

Visual defects

Visual defects should be understood, and one more list may be helpful.

1. Loss of visual field (hemianopia).
2. Difficulty in recognition (agnosia).
3. Inability to channel input (inattention).
4. Visuospatial disturbance.
5. Visual scanning (e.g. series of letters given, failure to pick out all 'O's).
6. Visual spanning (more complex instructions, e.g. cancel out 'D' when it occurs after 'E').

Neglect of half of space must be distinguished from visual loss of field.

DISORDERS OF SPEECH: A BREAKDOWN IN COMMUNICATION

Careful assessment of problems in communication is so important it should be undertaken by a specialist: the speech therapist. However, the problems that may occur should also be much better understood by other therapists and by the lay public. Believing this, I asked a senior speech therapist, Sandra Jackson Anderson, to write a report that other therapists and the lay public could understand, on the disabilities involved in speech disorders after stroke. This report (Jackson Anderson 1987) has helped many people and I have her permission to repeat it here.

INTRODUCTION

Probably one of the most appalling aspects of a stroke is that, for a few unfortunate patients, it can disrupt normal means of communication. Depending on the degree of severity, the patient may lose the power to understand speech, to read, to write and to communicate through words. One day to be healthy and the next to be paralysed is in itself an appalling experience, but to find also that you have no means of communicating must be terrifying. The stroke patient whose speech has not been affected is able to ask all the questions for which he must have answers. Why did it happen? Will it happen again? What can you do for me? What does the future hold? In so doing he is able to talk about his problems and alleviate his fears. The stroke patient who cannot speak often does not have these questions answered; he has no-one with whom to share his worries.

Immediately after the stroke he will feel very isolated, possibly depressed and even aggressive. Therefore, it is of the utmost importance that early on he is told what has happened and what we can hope for in the future. We must all be sensitive to his needs and anticipate the questions for which he must have answers. Although he cannot speak, or in some cases even understand, he is still the person he was before and should be treated as such. All those who have any dealings with him must explain what is being done for him and why. Even when we, the helpers, know that his ability to understand has been affected, we must still explain things to him slowly and clearly.

In the early days, the speech therapist may want to give intensive therapy herself, for at this stage it is often a job for the specialist. Only after the initial stages may she involve others in the direct treatment programme. However, that by no means implies that everyone else is redundant. Exercises alone do not bring back speech: rehabilitating the desire to communicate is the most important thing, and that is something which everyone must be involved in.

Never assume that because a patient is dumb he is also deaf for language. Never hold conversations around him: he must always be included no matter how severe his language problem. He has enough feelings of isolation within his own head without adding to them, and he needs all the support, communication and language stimulation that we can give.

Because he may feel isolated, it is essential that he is not isolated from language. He needs normal conversation, albeit one-sided. However, this conversation may need to be modified according to the type of communication problem which the patient has. Therefore, an attempt will be made here to describe the different communication problems that may follow a stroke and the best way to approach them.

WHAT ARE THE COMMUNICATION PROBLEMS?

The names given to disorders of communication following a stroke can be listed under three main headings: dysphasia, dyspraxia and dysarthria.

1. Dysphasia. There are two basic types of dysphasia: *receptive* and *expressive*. With this problem, the patient's language function has been reduced due to damage to the speech centres in the brain. He may be unable to understand speech and therefore also cannot speak logically; or he may be unable to find the correct sound or words for speech even if his understanding has not been affected.

*2. **Dyspraxia.*** This is generally found in conjunction with dysphasia. The patient may be able to select the correct word from his brain, but the lips and tongue will not coordinate properly to form the letters.

These two problems, dysphasia and dyspraxia, are, in the majority of cases, associated with a right-sided paralysis. This is because it is the left side of the brain which controls language, and it is that side of the brain which has been damaged.

*3. **Dysarthria.*** This is normally found in patients with a left-sided paralysis, and hence there is usually no language difficulty. The problem is purely at mouth level. The muscles are weak and because of this the speech is slurred and unintelligible. However, it should be noted that all patients with left-sided weakness do not necessarily suffer from dysarthria.

For the sake of clarity, these three disorders will be described separately, but it must be remembered that occasionally there can be a combination of speech disorders within the one person. That, however, can be fairly complex and is best described to all who care for the patient by the speech therapist who assesses him.

DYSPHASIA

RECEPTIVE DYSPHASIA

This is the most severe communication disorder. The patient's language as a whole – understanding, speaking, reading and writing – has been drastically reduced. For better understanding, the reason for this reduction can once more be subdivided under two headings: language input and language output.

Language input. The patient may understand very little of what is said to him. A good example of this problem will be demonstrated if you can imagine that you know a foreign language, e.g. French, in that you have attained a basic vocabulary and understand at no more than a fairly intermediate and limited level, and someone starts speaking to you. You would know that he was speaking French, you would be able to pick up the occasional word and perhaps get the gist of the conversation, but you would be unable to comprehend fully what was being said. This is perhaps the best way to imagine a receptive dysphasia, but this may only apply after the patient has recovered a little. In the dark days, immediately after the stroke, he may not realize that he has a language deficit and therefore may not be listening. Quite often the patient thinks that he is understanding, and that he is speaking perfectly logically. He may do what he thinks you have just asked him to do and then be surprised to find you shaking your head in disagreement. Likewise, he may become frustrated if you do not obey his commands or answer the questions which he believes he is asking. It is not difficult to imagine how totally bewildering these early days must be.

Language output. This can take several forms; the patient can be speechless and on the whole totally oblivious to language, or he can have a recurrent utterance, i.e. one word which he repeats over and over again, such as 'do – do – do'. Sometimes it may sound like speech because the patient may use the inflexion and intonation of speech but, if you listen closely, it may be nonsense, letters and sounds all mixed up, as, for example, 'bubble toe swarmer me'. Lastly the patient may be speaking in English words, but the content is often meaningless and there may be no grammatical form, e.g. 'may with house been was the are'. This is called 'jargon'.

Assessment of the patient's level of understanding

The most important thing to do initially, with a receptive dysphasia, is to ask the speech therapist to assess. This will show just how much the patient is understanding because, quite often, the level of understanding can be deceiving. As has been previously stated, the patient is still the same person as he was before. He is not demented or confused, he knows where he is and what is being done for him, and, in the early days in hospital, he may need to use very little language comprehension because there is so much visual stimulation with visual cues.

For example, a normal morning routine may start with the nurse bringing the patient a basin of water and saying: 'Get your facecloth and soap'. He does this, not necessarily because he understands what the nurse has said, but because it is the logical thing to do. She may then produce a shaving mirror and say: 'Get your razor'. (NB: An electric razor should be provided if the patient is using the nonpreferred hand.) Again he may do this because it is the next logical action in a chain of events. He may then be given his clothes, and here again, language comprehension may not be essential because he knows which garments to put on, albeit he may need help. So, on he may go to physiotherapy which is essentially physical, involving a great deal of gesture and visual cues. Here also, the need for language comprehension may be minimal. (Frequently in the early days of his second year, the human infant will carry out meaningful actions as a result of visual stimulation with visual cues, while his understanding of language is still limited.)

Next, the patient may go on to speech therapy. (In this case it is to be hoped that he does.) The speech therapist may discover that he can comprehend very little, and even finds difficulty in comprehending and obeying one simple command, e.g. 'Give me the pen', because she has taken away all visual cues and is making him rely solely on language. When she reports this information to the team who care for him, they may be astonished. The nurse may say that, although he cannot speak, he understood her perfectly that morning and did everything she asked. However, if the nurse had gone through the procedure in reverse, she might have got a very different reaction. For example, if she had gone to the patient and simply said: 'I am going to bring you a basin of water and a shaving mirror, could you get your soap, towel and razor ready?', she might have returned to find that he had done nothing because he had not understood; or that he had done something bizarre such as producing his dirty washing, because he had put a different interpretation on what she had said, perhaps from getting the gist of washing but not the full meaning.

Thus it can be seen how important gesture and nonverbal cues are to communication. It is also very important to realize the value of gesture in the early days. The use of gesture reduces frustration and is a necessary means of communication. However, as the patient becomes stronger, he must be made to listen to language and to interpret verbal as well as nonverbal messages.

With a receptive dysphasia, the speech therapist is primarily interested in finding out how much language the patient is understanding, and she has various assessments which she uses to ascertain this. She is looking for the answers to the following questions: Is her patient able to comprehend one simple sentence, or can he manage to understand two or more concepts at once? For how long can he concentrate? How accurate is his recent memory?

Communicating with the receptive dysphasic patient

When the speech therapist has discovered the level at which the language breakdown is occurring, she can then advise the relatives on the best way in which to communicate with the patient. Going back to the earlier example of someone speaking French, imagine how much easier it would be if, instead of speaking the language fluently, it was spoken slowly and simply. This would make it much easier to follow. So it is for the receptive dysphasic. In this case, to some extent, the patient's own language is now foreign to him.

Concentration and memory may also be reduced and dysphasic patients may be unable to cope with more than one concept at a time. For example, suppose the patient is given four questions in one quick sentence: 'It's a lovely day, isn't it? Would you like a cup of tea? Shall I move you over to the window to have it? Would you like to go to the toilet first?' Here, his brain has to process these four questions that are tossed at him in rapid succession before he produces an answer. In general, this would be too much for the patient with receptive problems to cope with. He cannot cope for the following reasons:

a. Language comprehension: too much language all at once.
b. Concentration: too many words and questions to be interpreted; he may lose interest.
c. Memory: he may forget one of the questions in his effort to interpret one of the others.

The above is perhaps a slightly exaggerated example, but hopefully it illustrates how not to speak to such a patient. Therefore, how should you speak to him? First, make sure you have his full attention; don't be afraid to touch his ear and say: 'Listen'. Then, very simply, one theme at a time, speak slowly and clearly. 'Would you like a cup of tea?' Give him plenty of time to interpret the question and indicate his answer. Then go on: 'Would you like to go to the toilet?' Again give him plenty of time. Lastly, without rushing: 'Would you like to sit by the window?'.

These essential rules apply to all receptive dysphasic patients:

1. Get the patient's attention.
2. Speak slowly and clearly.
3. Only offer one idea or question per sentence.

This sounds fairly simple, but it is probably one of the most difficult things to put into practice. Remember that the patient is still the same person as he was before and most adults would be highly insulted to have you 'spell it out in words of one syllable'. So, while the theory behind this is very easy to understand, putting it into practice can be very difficult. Obviously, if you sound condescending or childish when you speak to him, your patient may be even more frustrated, feeling that you are treating him as if he is daft when he knows he is still very normal. This is what must be guarded against very carefully.

The treatment programme for the patient with receptive dysphasia

As always, the speech therapist will assess the patient and plan a treatment programme. However, unlike the other speech problems in which the programme can be carried out jointly between therapists, relatives and nurses, the therapist may feel that if the problem is sufficiently severe, he may need treatment by the expert all the time. Therefore, after assessment, she may advise the relatives on the patient's level of understanding and how best to communicate with him, as has been previously described, but she may wish to carry out all the direct therapy herself. A receptive dysphasia is a very complex problem and in the early days is really best handled by the expert alone.

When the speech therapist has made the patient aware of his problems, and he knows what he must do to facilitate better language comprehension, then she may wish to enlist the help of others.

Always with a receptive problem, the starting point is input. Until this problem has been dealt with there can be no meaningful output. Were the problem to be approached the other way round and the output level tackled first, you could perhaps get the patient to name objects quite happily after you had done so. For example, you might teach him to say 'bed', but he would not be able to apply it in context if he felt tired. He would merely be repeating it parrot fashion. Also, to start work at this level would mean that you were rewarding with praise a response which you should really be inhibiting.

If the patient is not understanding you, he is probably not understanding himself, and he may be unable to organize his thoughts into some logical pattern. Therefore, the speech therapist will train him to listen carefully to what is said to him, process this in his mind, and produce the appropriate response. This is the response which must be strongly rewarded with praise, not the utterance, albeit correct, of an inappropriately used word.

In fact, the speech therapist will spend very little time on the patient's speech output in these early days. Her main concern will be to get him to begin listening and comprehending. The response for which she is aiming is normally a gestural one, in that she will give him a simple command, e.g. 'Pick up the pen'. He will have to listen carefully, interpret the message and perform the appropriate action, thus showing that he has comprehended. She may also work on reading, this too being an input task. This does not mean repeating after the therapist the word which is written. At this stage of therapy this word would only be a meaningless response. Here it means matching the appropriate written word to an object or picture which it describes. Work must therefore be done intensively on input, because the patient may then be able to use the words which he has in a meaningful way.

One of the main output problems with receptive dysphasics is that, where they have to be taught to listen to you, they likewise have to be taught to listen to themselves. They may believe that they are communicating with you and may not realize that they are producing jargon. Again, this is something that they must be made aware of. They have to be encouraged to listen to their own speech, check their own output and realize when they are speaking jargon.

From childhood we have been able to comprehend and speak automatically, not really consciously listening to either the input or the output. After a stroke, as described here, this is no longer automatic, and listening must be taught as a new skill. However, once that skill has been learned and the patient realizes that sometimes he doesn't understand and doesn't speak logically, then he is on the road to recovery. Perhaps his language will never return completely, but, with the help of the speech therapist and the care of the family, he can hopefully reach a level of communication which is adequate for his everyday needs and which reduces frustration.

EXPRESSIVE DYSPHASIA

With this problem, language and communication are again greatly reduced. Reading, writing and speaking are affected but comprehension for the greater part is intact. Hence, the patient can understand what is being said, and is generally able to form a logical response in his own mind, but cannot find the correct words to put his response into speech.

There are several ways in which this problem presents itself. In the most severe form, the patient may be virtually speechless, perhaps only able to say 'yes' and 'no', and these words may be used, as is often the case with all dysphasias, inconsistently and inappropriately. The patient may also have a recurrent utterance, i.e. he may continue to say the same meaningless phrase, e.g. 'comes and been' every time he attempts speech. Patients with not quite so much damage may be able to communicate in single words and short phrases, their ability to produce grammatical sentences having been reduced. Finally, in its less severe form, the patient may be able to speak almost normally, but may occasionally have difficulty in finding the words he wants.

Word-finding difficulty is common to all patients with an expressive dysphasia; it is as if their mind momentarily goes blank and they have really to think and search to find the words. The other problem for these patients is that when they produce a word it may be the wrong one. For example, they may mean to say 'television' but instead produce 'chair'; or, if they do say 'television', which may be the correct response, all subsequent responses may be 'television': the needle has a habit of getting stuck! This can be tremendously frustrating because the patient with the purely expressive problem, as you would expect, has a greater ability to hear himself than the receptively damaged patient. Thus, his own responses are often as frustrating to him as they are to the listener.

As already stressed, the problem affects language as a whole. Therefore, as with speech, his reading and writing will also be affected to a greater or lesser extent. The patient may be able to read and comprehend simple words, or he may be able to read the newspaper headlines and possibly to read and comprehend a short paragraph or newspaper article. Writing, as this is an output task, is always much poorer than reading and you will find that writing ability generally falls far short of reading comprehension.

Assessment of patients with expressive dysphasia

When assessing these patients, the speech therapist is going to look firstly at comprehension. Although this is an expressive dysphasia, there are often comprehension problems in the early days. These are not necessarily due to language loss, but to fatigue and general exhaustion. Having a stroke takes a tremendous amount out of a person, and the patient may quite simply be far too tired to concentrate on what is being said. Therefore, the speech therapist must assess how long he can concentrate for. She may even decide that 5 or 10 minutes' language stimulation is all that he can cope with at any one time. This assessment of therapy time is something which applies to all the communication problems, not just the expressive one. Hopefully, as he gets stronger, his tolerance to therapy will improve.

Once the speech therapist has assessed any input problem, she will look at the main problem which in this case is output. She will want to know the exact level at which the patient's language breaks down. How much speech does he have? If there is no propositional (self-elicited or meaningful) speech, can he be stimulated to produce it? Is he communicating with a few words? Is he using words or sentences? When she has found the breakdown level, she will want to look at it in detail. What words is he producing? How often does he have difficulty in finding words? How often does he find a wrong word by mistake? If he is producing sentences, at which level does his grammar break down? Is he using mainly phrases or sentences? Is he using prepositions, tenses, etc correctly? The therapist will also test reading comprehension. She must know at which level (words, sentences or paragraphs) reading comprehension fails. Lastly she will assess meaningful writing; however, as this is an output task, it will probably not be beyond the one word stage, at most, initially.

Treatment programme for the patient with expressive dysphasia

With these questions answered, the treatment programme is started at the appropriate breakdown level, and follows a normal developmental pattern from there on, working on speaking, reading and writing exercises. As with a receptive dysphasic, the aim is not to get the patient to produce words which are meaningless, but to produce good propositional speech. This is achieved by language stimulation. For example, you would not say to the patient: 'Chair. . . you say it . . . chair!'. This is because, as with the receptive dysphasic, you would perhaps get a meaningless parroted response. It is therefore better to stimulate him by visual and auditory means to produce the correct response. So, the correct way to elicit the word 'chair' would be to say: 'Chair, you sit on a. . .' and, hopefully, the patient would say the word, his brain having received the correct stimulus. You are giving him a cue and this is the best way to help his word-finding difficulty.

General communication with these patients is easier, because, unlike the receptive dysphasics, their own thought processes, etc are relatively intact. They know what they want, and by process of elimination, pointing, gesture and/or use of single words, they are often able to express their needs. So, on a basic day-to-day level, it is less frustrating. However, their main frustration arises from the fact that they are aware of what is going on around them. They are listening to conversation and, if involved in a conversation, may want to add a point, contradict what is being said, or crack a joke. Imagine the feelings of an expressive dysphasic patient if he opens his mouth to make a joke and either nothing or meaningless words result. People immediately want to help with what he is wanting to say but it's not funny any more. Or, imagine the immense frustration of having to listen to a conversation with which you disagree violently, and being unable to state your point of view, or indeed, due to paralysis, being unable to get up and walk away from the source of frustration.

Therefore, with an expressive dysphasic patient (indeed all patients with problems of communication) it is essential that you are not only sensitive to the patient's everyday needs, but also to his emotional needs. The best help can sometimes be to imagine yourself in his position, and thereby sharpen your own sensitivity to his communicative needs.

DYSPRAXIA

This problem generally occurs along with dysphasia, either receptive or expressive. It is a complex problem and one which can be difficult to describe. It may even affect the whole body, limbs as well as mouth. However for the sake of clarity, the dyspraxia discussed in this section will be coupled with an expressive dysphasia.

'Dyspraxia' is the term used for difficulty in performing voluntary movements, occurring because of damage to sensory and motor areas of the brain. The word comes from the Greek *praxis,* 'doing'. An understanding of this problem is essential if an intelligent approach is to be made to rehabilitation. Where it concerns the body as a whole it may result in failure to draw coherently, failure to deal effectively with or manipulate objects and failure to integrate acts into sequence. The only way to tackle the problem from a physical point of view is to follow the lines already described, going right back to the beginning and working through the infant patterns of motor and sensory development, remembering that a successful outcome may take many weeks (or even months) of treatment.

Where this problem occurs in the area of speech, extra help will be needed. It may often go undiagnosed and unnoticed but, in this case, leads to failure in speech rehabilitation. Therefore another simple example is given below as an aid to understanding.

If you ask the patient to stick out his tongue, a receptive dysphasic may not do it because he does not understand the command and a dysarthric patient may not do it because his muscles are too weak. A dyspraxic patient would:

a. understand the command, and
b. attempt to perform the movement, but somewhere between comprehending and performing there is a breakdown, and instead of the tongue coming out, it may go to the back of his mouth. He has clearly understood but his mouth will not do what he wants it to.

The assessment of this difficulty can really only be carried out by the speech therapist, as it is very similar in appearance to an expressive dysphasia and the defining line is not always clear. There is generally a language loss with this problem in that the patient may have a moderate expressive dysphasia, but his communication difficulty may be severe because of dyspraxia. Part of his problem will be due to word-finding difficulty, i.e. the word he wants does not come readily to mind and he really has to search for it. However, it may also be partly due to the dyspraxia; he does not find the correct word in his brain, knows what he wants to say, tries to say it, but his brain does not coordinate with the tongue and the lips and the wrong sound comes out.

So, as you can see, the dyspraxic patient, like the dysphasic patient, may be producing wrong sounds or words and may also have a recurrent utterance, but the neurological reasons are very different.

As previously stated, this problem is generally found coupled with dysphasia. Therefore the patient's reading and writing are affected. His reading level may be slightly higher because there is probably less language loss than with a pure expressive dysphasia. However this is not the case with writing. Again, because of language loss, but also because (as with the mouth) the brain may not be coordinating with the motor performance (this time the arm), writing may be equally poor. Therefore, to all intents and purposes, these two problems (dysphasia and dyspraxia) are very similar in the picture which they represent.

When the speech therapist has diagnosed a dyspraxia, the treatment would probably have a dual purpose. She would treat the dysphasia as described and she would also give exercises to help improve the coordination of the lips, tongue, etc. Relaxation is also an important factor; therapy sessions should be as stress-free as possible because the more tense these patients become the harder it is for them to coordinate. Family and nurses can help by offering the same kind of treatment they should give to the patient with expressive dysphasia. The patient can understand, so speak to him normally, stimulate his responses but don't get him to repeat unless the speech therapist specially asks for this as part of the treatment programme.

In very few cases, it is possible to find an almost pure dyspraxia, i.e. language involvement is minimal. These patients may therefore still be able to read books and may perhaps be able to write single propositional words, which they can use as a dual means of communication along with whatever speech they have. However this is not a very common disorder, and is best described to you by the speech therapist who diagnoses it.

DYSARTHRIA

With this problem, as previously stated, there is no language loss. Generally speaking, the patient can read and write, he knows or understands what you are saying and in return will speak in perfectly logical, well-formed sentences which, however, due to muscle weakness, are often barely intelligible.

Characteristically, speech is slow, slurred, monotonous and often nasal. This is due to weakness of the lips, tongue and soft palate. Hence, you may also find that the patient has difficulty in eating and is prone to drooling, which is a tremendous social handicap and which can further lead to his feeling isolated and inadequate.

When the speech therapist assesses the dysarthric patient she is going to look first at the sounds he is making. She must find out the following:

1. What sounds can he make?
2. What sounds can he approximate?
3. What sounds are lost?

She will then find out if his breathing pattern is accurate for speech: does he have enough breath to raise his voice, or to speak a sentence? This leads to other questions. For example, at what pace does he speak, is it abnormally fast or slow? Is his speech pretty monotonous, or is he managing some intonation to colour it? In other words, does he produce the normal rise and fall of the voice when speaking?

Once these questions have all been answered, the speech therapist will decide upon a treatment programme which, as always, can be carried out by nurses and/or relatives as advised by her.

Treatment would involve exercises to improve movement in the lips, tongue and palate, and here the physiotherapist can often give her expert advice. Together she and the speech therapist may devise a suitable scheme of exercises that will help to overcome the problem. A small block of wet ice may be used to good effect to massage affected facial muscles. For ice treatment and for exercise the physiotherapist thinks in terms of muscle direction, and she may use her fingers or a wooden spatula to give any desired assistance or resistance to any movement.

The exercise offered jointly by the speech therapist and the physiotherapist may include some, or all, of the following suggestions. Exercises may be given unilaterally or bilaterally (or both) and, if necessary, will include eyebrows, eyes, nose and mouth. The therapist may use her fingers and thumbs to depress the eyebrows and then ask her patient to raise them, giving assistance or resistance as necessary. He may be asked to screw up his eyes while she gives resistance to the movement, to sniff against mild resistance given when she closes his nostrils with finger and thumb, and to smile and then to purse his lips with assistance and against resistance. He may be asked to suck against resistance offered by two wooden spatulas which are held inside his mouth with a mild lateral pull to give a wide grin. The tongue will be exercised against resistance offered by the wooden spatula and jaw movements are practised. The help of a mirror for facial exercises may be necessary.

Breathing exercises will be given, and exercises to improve the accuracy of the speech sounds. Any intonation exercises given to reduce the monotony of the patient's speech will include phrasing exercises. Using short phrases instead of long sentences obviously improves clarity, and reminds the patient to speak slowly and clearly.

Therapy for the dysarthric patient can therefore be undertaken jointly by the speech therapist and the physiotherapist.

When you have been advised about exercises, it is essential that they are practised every day. With a little effort, speech can become more intelligible and general quality of voice will improve and become more pleasant.

With some patients there may be drooling and difficulty in swallowing food. Here the speech therapist may be able to demonstrate some techniques which can be employed to reduce the problem. However, one thing to be remembered is that swallowing saliva may no longer be automatic. If there is a facial paralysis and weakness of muscles of the mouth, the swallowing reflex may be reduced and the patient may be unaware of saliva gathering in his mouth. So, having someone to remind him that he needs to swallow is often more helpful than giving him a handkerchief to wipe his mouth. He can often be taught to remember to swallow.

The next point applies to all stroke patients with communication problems, but especially to those who are dysarthric. Dentures and hearing aids must be examined. Always, after a stroke, have hearing aids checked to ensure that they are working efficiently, and indeed it may be advisable to have the hearing retested. Likewise, consult the dentist. Find out if the existing dentures still fit or would they benefit from a reline to make them fit better. Perhaps the patient may require a completely new set. Make sure that maximum benefit is being received from these aids.

Lastly, as there is generally no language involvement, the dysarthric patient may still be able to write. However, in a few patients, writing may be difficult for various reasons and some retraining by the speech therapist may be necessary. Writing can often be used along with speech as a dual means of communication, and some severely dysarthric patients may find writing to be a necessary alternative.

POINTS TO REMEMBER

The following should be borne in mind when communicating with the patient:

1. Remember the golden rule which has been stressed throughout this whole section: speak to the patient as you would speak to any normal intelligent adult.
2. Remember that with the dysphasic patient, reading and writing are also affected. Therefore, *never* give a patient paper and a pencil and ask him to write down what he is trying to say. This only causes frustration and depression; remember it is language as a whole which is affected.
3. Likewise, don't give him the usual load of paperbacks and magazines which are so much a part of hospital visiting. In the early days he may become even more depressed when he realizes that his reading ability is greatly reduced.

However, as he becomes stronger and more able to cope with his disability it is advisable to restart his daily paper and favourite magazine. Even if he can only read the headlines and look at the pictures, he is becoming reorientated and will benefit from the language stimulation. At this stage you can also read out short articles to him, letting him follow the words with you.

4. Arithmetic is also generally affected. So, don't trust him to pay the milkman unless you leave the exact money!

5. For all speech-damaged patients, dysarthric, dyspraxic and dysphasic, another essential rule applies: never stop and talk unless you have time to listen. If you are busy, just wave or shout a cheery 'Hello!' Communication with these patients is slow and it is obviously more frustrating for them if you stop to chat briefly and have to leave without finding out what they are saying.

6. Communication charts must be mentioned. There are two or three types available. These are charts with pictures of articles the patient may need, e.g. toilet, spectacles, etc. We have found that these are of little value to a dysphasic patient, and are only really of any use with the dysarthric patient. The dysphasic patient may be unable to select the appropriate picture due to damaged mental processing, or, as these patients often have visual problems, they may be unable to see or recognize the pictures due to an excess of visual stimulus. Therefore, these charts, if used inappropriately, can be a further source of frustration and so the advice of the therapist should be sought before introducing them.

7. Positioning is also very important during speech therapy; indeed as it is 24 hours a day following a stroke. The patient should be positioned carefully in the correct chair with a table at a suitable working height as already described (see Fig. 17) and the hemiplegic arm correctly supported. The therapist sits on his affected side or immediately in front of him. Speech therapy requires tremendous concentration from the patient and if spasticity and pain develop, his power of concentration will be reduced. Correct positioning before commencing treatment is essential. The therapist's room should be suitably quiet.

8. Finally, we have not included any specific exercises for the dysphasic and dyspraxic patients because this is virtually impossible without knowing the individual patient and his problem. The differential diagnosis between dyspraxia and receptive and expressive dysphasia is a job for the speech therapist, who, having carried out an assessment, will advise on exercises which will be appropriate for the individual patient. To perform 'speech exercises' with a patient who has not been professionally assessed is of little value and these exercises can, if wrongly administered, lead yet again to frustration.

Sandra Jackson Anderson

OTHER PROBLEMS TO BE SOLVED

There are still some physical problems which must be discussed. To be aware of some of these is to take preventative action, but in any case, problems are there to be solved.

THE HEMIPLEGIC SHOULDER

Hemiplegic shoulder problems have already been discussed with the introduction to the use of pressure splints. The untreated stiff painful shoulder, if it has developed, will lead to permanent disability of the hemiplegic arm. When dealing with the hemiplegic shoulder the general rule is to maintain mobility with outward rotation of the joint and a freely moving scapula which will slide round the chest wall. However, if this mobility has already been lost, make use of the arm stability offered by the inflatable pressure splint and manually mobilize the upper trunk and shoulder, at all times maintaining the vital outward rotation of the shoulder joint. If the rules for mobilizing the stiff painful shoulder (given earlier in this text) are carefully followed all should be well.

LOSS OF THE MEMORY OF MOVEMENT

In the days immediately following a stroke the patient's brain will readily both forget established movement patterns and adopt new, abnormal ones, which are largely dictated by spasticity. This can quickly constitute a major barrier to successful rehabilitation as it is enormously difficult to reverse this process. Loss of kinaesthetic memory is a negative sign. Man can only perform movements which he has experienced before. There seems to be a complete wiping out of memory and it is useless to expect to carry out a movement with the sound side and imitate with the affected side. The brain will not connect the two.

The patient must relearn the feeling of movement; it is no wonder that sensory loss can present such a rehabilitation problem. The case for stepping up sensory input has been given; now the patient needs repetition, over and over again in movement patterns, but the latter must be performed with sustained pressure support maintaining inhibiting patterns. For the realization of a movement you have to make it possible. The patient is bound to coordinate wrong movement unless he has the memory of correct movement. Treatment consists of enabling him to remember the normal movement. He may be in a vicious circle of abnormal input and output, he may even be paralysed, and treatment must break this vicious circle.

Treatment should begin early before this becomes a major problem. Step up sensory input and give repetition over and over again. However, this must be the rule for all stroke rehabilitation, with emphasis on the need to start treatment early.

I find that loss of the memory of movement is much less of a problem since I started to use pressure techniques with inhibiting patterns and increased sensory input. The whole concept of treatment is based on the need to restore normal postural tone and a normal postural reflex mechanism. Normal movement patterns must not be lost.

Summary

The points concerning loss of the memory of movement may be summed up as follows:

1. There are positive and negative signs. Too much movement, where the patient overshoots his target, is a positive sign. Loss of function is a negative sign.
2. The brain forgets established movement patterns.
3. The brain quickly adopts new abnormal patterns.
4. This rapidly erects a major barrier to rehabilitation.
5. Loss of kinaesthetic memory seems to be a complete wiping out of memory.
6. It is of no use to perform movements with the sound side and then mimic with the affected side. The brain will not connect the two.
7. Treatment must be early, stepping up sensory input and giving a great deal of repetition, starting with passive and inhibitory controlled movement patterns and advancing to active and inhibitory controlled movement patterns. Pressure splints are used to give stability and to control tonal flow, diverting it into inhibitory patterns.
8. Attempt to get the patient's full concentration and ask him to 'think the movement' as you perform it passively. Attempt to get his memory to retain the normal pattern and gradually let him take over, going through the stages of active assisted to active movement.
9. A quiet room will be necessary for this kind of treatment.
10. Again, it is essential to base the recovery programme on motor development patterns.

EXTENSOR SPASTICITY IN THE LEG

This will often be found if correct practices in rehabilitation have not been established early after the onset of the stroke. However, once again with the intervention of pressure splint techniques, reversing this abnormal tonal pattern is possible. Rehabilitation stages should be understood.

1. Teach and use inhibiting positioning at all times.
2. Give passive movements in inhibiting patterns, but remember that the positioning of the physiotherapist's hands is of extreme importance. For example, she must not place a hand under the forepart of the foot and her other hand behind his knee; this would only assist the thrust of the leg downwards into the unwanted extension. One hand should be placed firmly under the patient's heel while the therapist's other hand will direct the movement into inward rotation with flexion of the hip.
3. Change passive movements into assisted active movements as rehabilitation advances, and work towards unassisted voluntary movement.
4. Use placing and movement in inhibiting patterns.
5. Use leg gaiter training as already described to encourage weightbearing through the heel of a correctly positioned foot, distributing weight up through a semiflexed knee to an inwardly rotated hip. This will inhibit the strong extensor thrust of gluteus maximus and increase tone in the low tonal pattern of flexion.

6. The use of a rocking chair, provided careful inhibiting positioning is used, will be much more beneficial than the use of a static chair. With careful foot positioning the patient will use his leg within an inhibiting pattern with each rock of the chair *provided he pushes through his heels* and not through his toes. He may need a footstool to achieve this. A solid wooden box is best. Positioning (as in all instances) must include arm positioning.
Note: A footboard for bed rest must never be used. If a footboard is used, the front part of the patient's foot will push against it, bringing in an extensor response and increasing the unwanted extensor spasticity.

THE INVERTED SPASTIC FOOT

This is frequently the result of lack of the correct early care. It is not a problem where rocking chair and gaiter training for the leg are used in early rehabilitation.

Late treatment

This should be carried out as follows:

1. Go back to the beginning and check recovery in the lower trunk and hip. Any weakness or spasticity in this area must be dealt with.
2. As suggested above, use the rocking chair with careful positioning of the hip and foot.
3. Use weightbearing in inhibiting positions. Study the correct foot position as illustrated in Figure 26B and apply the leg gaiter to maintain the semiflexed knee. Use the gaiter training exercises, as in Chapter 4, for extensor spasticity in the leg.
4. When doing mat work, bridging is useful but inhibit strongly over the foot. This should be achieved by the physiotherapist's bending up the toes, particularly the great toe, with weight bearing through the heel.
5. Use sitting to standing from a low stool with the affected foot carefully positioned. Remember in sitting to standing the sound foot should be just in front of the affected foot, the foot in front taking less weight than the foot behind. Use the long arm splint to take care of associated reactions.
6. Do not use a rigid foot splint; use a lively splint, if any. At this late stage in rehabilitation, which can be classed as a 'rescue job', I would recommend the Air-stirrup Ankle Training Brace as marketed by Aircast, if any is to be used. However, it is of no use to tackle the problem from the wrong end. Full recovery will only taken place if it comes from the hip downwards (see point 1). However, the antispasticity pattern of the total hip to foot must be maintained at all times, and carefully used for all exercise routines, particularly for weight-bearing, with the ankle protected against increasing spasticity and undue strain while recovery takes place from above downwards. I have found point 3, above, of particular value in this situation. Also a lateral raise of 1 cm (0.5 inches) sloping inwards, on the outside of firm supporting footwear, can be very useful. The raise must level off to nil halfway across the sole. The most severe case of the inverted spastic foot I have ever encountered responded well to the recommended wedge on the sole of a boot which laced up above the ankle,

with the addition of the Air-stirrup Ankle Training Brace worn inside the boot.

LONG-TERM FLACCIDITY OF THE ARM

Refer back to the section on the use of pressure splints (Ch. 4).

OEDEMA OF THE HAND

Refer back to the section on the use of pressure splints (Ch. 4).

THE 'PUSHER SYNDROME'

The 'pusher syndrome', or the persistent lateral lean, presents a situation which many find difficult to treat. However, far from being a severe complication which interferes with satisfactory rehabilitation, it can be used to give positive assistance in the treatment programme.

The average stroke patient cannot and will not transfer his weight across to the affected side of his body. He will move from sitting to standing, compensating for his loss of function by using his sound side. This means that he stands up taking all his weight only on his unaffected side, using his hemiplegic leg as no more than a prop, toes in contact with the ground. Antigravity tone will usually develop at an alarming rate, giving the all too familiar picture of extensor spasticity as described above, all the way down from the hip to the inverted foot.

As recovery depends on re-establishing a balanced body with normal muscle tone, it is essential that he should aim to recover normal standing balance. To do this his advancing rehabilitation programme must use weightbearing through both sides of his body with inhibiting positions guarding against the onset (and ever-increasing problem) of spasticity. As the whole concept of treatment rests with the need to restore normal postural tone, the patient must be taught to transfer his weight over onto his affected side and then progress to trunk stability with even tonal distribution through both sides of his body. It sometimes takes many weeks of training before the patient is able to stand and transfer his weight across to his affected side, but this must be achieved.

The patient with the pusher syndrome presents with a totally opposite situation. Here, when the patient attempts to stand, he pushes strongly on his sound foot to stand up and, as he stands, all his weight is thrown across to his affected side in a dangerous lateral lean which his hemiplegic side cannot support. Even if he is fully supported on his affected side by a helper, she will not be able to cope with the demand made on her, particularly where the overweight patient is concerned. They may both end up on the floor. The pusher syndrome is usually a sign of severe sensory loss.

This apparently disastrous situation will be best turned to the patient's advantage in the following treatment sequence:

1. Early daily training in rolling is essential and should lead as soon as possible into rolling over and over right across a large floor space. For this routine the patient's hands will be clasped and held up above his head (see Fig. 12). It is vital to bombard proprioceptors and to stimulate reflex levels, particularly righting reflexes.
2. Mat work should include all head and neck routines, and trunk stabilizing, with stability given to the hemiplegic arm by a long arm pressure splint.
3. Daily training in standing balance should also start early. The Arjo Lift Walker presently found in many physiotherapy departments (see Fig. 48 and below) gives ideal patient support. Two therapists may also be required to assist the patient into standing, suitably positioned, and then to apply two gaiters, one on each leg. The gaiters must be positioned high up under the ischial tuberosities, with the zip fasteners running down the middle of the lateral aspect of the leg. The posterior section is inflated first in the usual way with mild flexion of the knees and the heel firmly on the floor. Finally, the anterior chamber is inflated minimally to stabilize pressure round the knee. Both gaiters are applied in this way. The hemiplegic arm should also be carefully positioned, in ulna border leaning, if possible. This is easily achieved where an Arjo Lift Walker is available, or a suitable standing table. The half-arm splint is used on the hemiplegic forearm, and both arms are positioned with the patient bearing weight through parallel forearms.
4. With the whole of the hemiplegic side of the body well supported with the stability offered by pressure splints, the patient is now fully bearing weight through his affected side which is positioned in inhibiting patterns. Without the pusher syndrome this can be very slow to be established. With the pusher syndrome it is quickly and easily established provided both legs are supported by leg gaiters and the pelvis is balanced.
5. Trunk stabilizing in standing is undertaken with the patient positioned as in point 4. Note that it is also essential to continue the daily sessions in rolling.

This shows how an apparently disastrous situation can be turned to the patient's advantage.

Note that where you are dealing with the pusher syndrome and the use of two gaiters, both feet remain firmly on the floor, and trunk training and all weight shifts are brought about by the physiotherapist and the demands she makes on her patient, by using both her hands to apply gentle and varying pressures.

FLEXOR WITHDRAWAL OF THE HEMIPLEGIC LEG

Flexor withdrawal of the hemiplegic leg where the hemiplegic leg goes into flexion and the patient stands only on his sound leg can present a problem. This is not a common condition but it does occur occasionally. As far as I know this has not been fully explained, but I have found it to occur in previously pinned hips or in association with pain in the lumbar region, and have thought it may be a withdrawal reflex.

If this problem does occur it must be met with a satisfactory rehabilitation approach and once again the inflatable gaiter is brought into use, but with a second and different method of application. As already described, the gaiter is wrapped round the leg and the zip fastener closed. The gaiter is carefully positioned as before, but the patient is lying comfortably supported on his back. In this second method of application, the anterior chamber is inflated first, to give firm support with the knee in extension. The posterior chamber is inflated next to give all-round stability to the knee, and the leg is in extension. The patient is then assisted into a standing position with both feet in a suitable weightbearing position. In this standing position, if it is found to be necessary, a second gaiter may be applied to the other leg to assist total stability and trunk training.

It will be readily understood that this second method of application of the leg gaiter must not be used on the much more usual tonal pattern, where the need is to inhibit antigravity tone and, in particular, the antigravity leg pattern which is mainly established by the strong action of gluteus maximus and hip extension, leading to total extension of the rest of the leg. Here, it is essential to use the first method where the posterior chamber of the splint is inflated first.

Again note that this is not a splint to be used for walking. As soon as you are satisfied that the splinted leg is correctly positioned the hemiplegic foot does not leave the floor. Standing exercises and weight shifts are brought about by movement of the sound leg.

Treated in this way I have not found the pusher syndrome or the flexor withdrawal problem to persist over a long period.

In all situations the tonal pattern in the arm must be carefully guarded and the build-up by associated reactions of excessive antigravity tone should be prevented wherever necessary by the application of the appropriate pressure splint while work takes place on the trunk and legs.

The Arjo Lift Walker

Figure 48 illustrates the Arjo Lift Walker which is not used as a 'walker' for the stroke patient. It is used with the brakes on and it does not move. With arm rests of adjustable height, it can be used to support parallel forearms, elbows immediately under the shoulders, or, with the arm rests lowered, it can be used to support an inhibited hand position with the patient leaning through both hands with straight elbows. Where necessary, inhibiting patterns are maintained with pressure splint support.

OTHER PROBLEMS OF WHICH THE THERAPIST SHOULD BE AWARE

Some of the problems that may be encountered in stroke treatment include: mild spasticity to severe spasticity; mild pain to severe pain; loss of confidence to a feeling of hopeless inadequacy, and low morale ranging from uninterested apathy to deep depression and withdrawal into complete isolation. It often

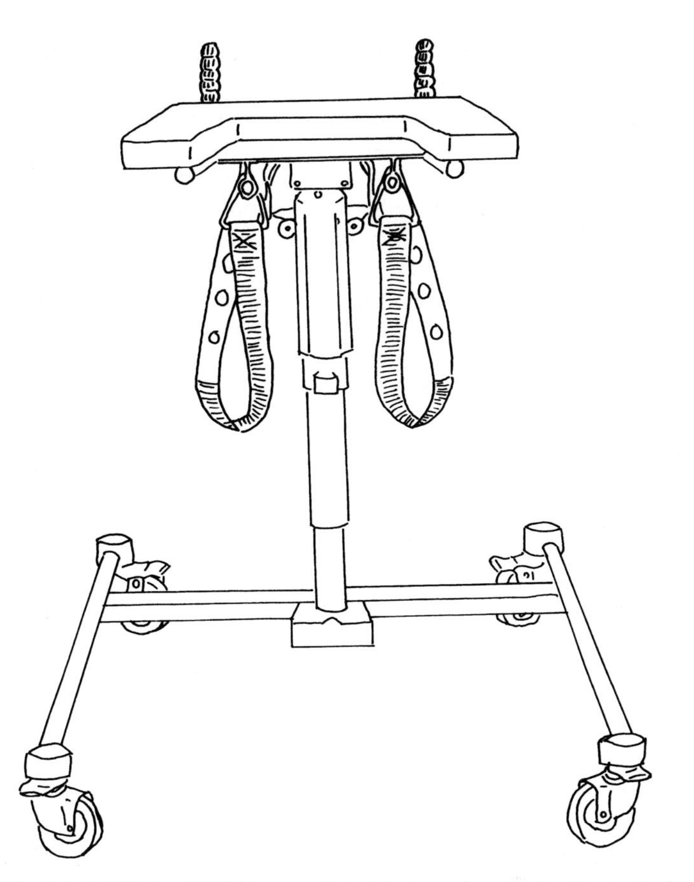

Fig. 48 The Arjo Lift Walker 214141, a most useful piece of apparatus in any stroke unit.

does not take many weeks for the stroke patient to produce some, if not all, of these symptoms, if no serious or worthwhile rehabilitation has been offered. We should not delude ourselves into believing that these are simply symptoms of any stroke, and moreover, symptoms that are to be expected after a stroke. They are not problems; they are symptoms of a problem, the problem being failure in so many cases to approach these unfortunate patients with a rehabilitation programme which raises the spirits, giving hope because it points in a meaningful way towards physical recovery. We need properly integrated stroke teams, with the different specialties working as one unit and for each patient, wherever possible, a family member should be included. I would like to quote from an occupational therapist who obviously understands this need (Eggers 1983):

> *Today, with specialisation, there are clear demarcations among the professions. Even so, there are points of contact and overlap because fundamentally all are striving to reach the same treatment goals. A well-functioning rehabilitation team is one where the transition of the patient from one mode to another is smooth.*

I am happy to be able to report that I have come across occupational therapists in various parts of the world who are successfully integrating the use of inflatable pressure splints into their care of stroke patients. Occupational therapists have much to offer and where physiotherapists, speech therapists and nurses work together as a united whole, we have the 'well-functioning rehabilitation team where the transition of the patient from one mode to another is smooth'. All work together for the good of the patient.

Constant repetition of any therapeutic exercise is a basic need in the restoration of motor control. The occupational therapist has the ability to motivate the patient by putting him in a situation where he can see a result each time he performs a stated exercise. Combining this with pressure splint techniques to control the distribution of muscle tone can have excellent results, e.g. with the patient where logic is missing.

CASE STUDY ON 35 ELDERLY PATIENTS

It took me 2 years to build just such a well-functioning rehabilitation team, as mentioned above, in a long-term hospital where many elderly patients were spending their last years. It was a wonderful study ground, turning up every conceivable problem and I stayed there for 10 years. During two of those years I carried out a single-patient case study of 35 elderly patients (Johnstone 1989). The results are presented here.

Criteria for entering study

These were:

1. severe disability
2. failure to rehabilitate elsewhere, and placed in long-term care
3. motor/sensory loss
4. other medical problems from mild to severe.

Aim of treatment

This was to reach a reasonable level of self-care and so be able to return to the community and leave long-term care.

Methods of treatment

These included the following:

1. Inhibiting positioning.
2. Movement into patterns which opposed spasticity patterns.
3. Sustained pressure used to maintain inhibiting patterns, controlling tonal flow with early mobility and intensive weightbearing.
4. Intermittent pressure for sensory input (40 mmHg for 3 seconds to 10 mmHg for 3 seconds, alternating for an average of 45 minutes twice daily).

Disabilities discovered by assessment tests

The patients fell into four groups.

a. Severe motor loss with spasticity, plus mild medical problems, was found in 15 patients.

b. Severe motor and sensory loss, plus mild medical problems, was found in 10 patients.
c. In five patients the disabilities mentioned in a. and b. were found, with the addition of more severe medical problems. These failed to rehabilitate.
d. In five patients the disabilities mentioned in a. and b. were found, with the addition of very severe medical problems. These died.

Outcome of study

These 35 cases were collected over 2 years. Of the patients, 25 returned to the community, five failed to rehabilitate and five patients died.

The rehabilitation time ranged from 3 months to 1 year.

The quality of life for the patient should never be forgotten. To rehabilitate is to restore lost or forfeited rights. Perhaps we ought to be comparing the cost of setting up efficient stroke units with the cost of keeping patients in long-term care for the rest of their days.

THE ASSESSMENT CHART

A stroke assessment chart ought to be used and yet it remains one of the most difficult treatment aids to produce. It is a treatment aid because treatment will not make a balanced all-purpose approach towards the problem of rehabilitating a whole person without careful assessment which will uncover all the problems. Assessment charts tend to be too brief and do not give an overall picture, or they tend to be too long (sometimes many pages) and it is impossible to see the state of a patient at a glance. It is necessary to attempt to draw up an assessment chart which not only gives a clear picture of the patient's motor and sensory disability, but which also acts as a progress report.

Figures 49–51 give a suggested layout for the assessment chart.

Figure 52 illustrates the first page of just such an assessment chart which shows the improvement in gross motor performance over a period of 5 months. One glance at this chart gives you a progress report. The assessment chart is stapled together with a fourth blank sheet for any further necessary comments. It is by no means the perfect assessment chart but it is offered with the following recommendations:

1. It covers most of the necessary data.
2. Therapists might be prepared to use it, assess its shortcomings and make improvements where necessary.

DRAWING UP AND USING AN ASSESSMENT CHART

The following points should be remembered:

1. Receptive and expressive ability cannot be assessed accurately immediately after a stroke. It may be some time before a high level of receptive disability is picked up. An early assessment can only be a snap assessment and the examiner must keep an open mind.

Name .... Age ....

Diagnosis .... Occupation ....

Date of onset .... Ward ....

Date of admission .... Date of discharge ....

Muscle tone

Are the limbs resistant to the following movements or are they heavy and abnormally relaxed?

	Date				
Arm: movement into recovery pattern plus elevation.					
Leg: movement into recovery pattern plus full flexion.					

(State: resistant or heavy = spastic or flaccid = S1, 2, 3 or F1, 2, 3.)

Gross motor performance

In bed	Date				
1. Roll from supine to right					
2. Roll from supine to left					
3. Bridging					
4. Roll to elbow propping					
5. Roll to sitting over edge of bed					
6. Sitting without use of hands					
7. Transfer from bed to chair					
In physiotherapy					
1. Rolling to prone lying					
2. Prone lying with forearm support					
3. Kneeling with forearm support					
4. Full kneeling to stand kneeling					
5. Crawling					
Balance					
1. In sitting					
2. In kneeling					
3. In standing					
Weight transfers					
1. Over affected hip in sitting					
2. Over affected hand in sitting					
3. Cross R leg over L in sitting					
4. Cross L leg over R in sitting					
5. Sitting to standing with hands clasped					
6. Over affected hip in standing					
7. Controlled walking					

Scale of grading: 3, unaided; 2, with minimal help; 1, with help; 0, impossible

Fig. 49 Assessment chart for stroke patients: page 1.

Record returning normal muscle tone

Grade 1–5   5 = Normal, associated reactions nil (see below)

Upper limb (supine)

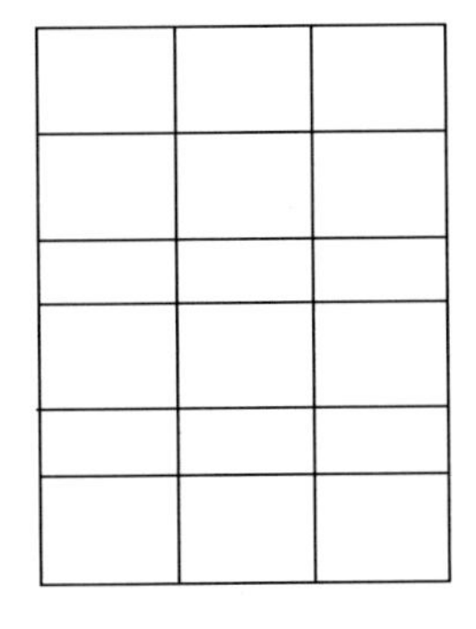

1. Patient holding extended arm in elevation, arm vertical, it having been placed there.
2. Lower the extended arm through abduction from elevation to horizontal.
3. Return.
4. With extended arm in elevation, bend elbow to touch top of head in supination.
5. Return in supination.
6. Hold extended arm in elevation, in lateral rotation, grasp and release.

Lower limb (supine)

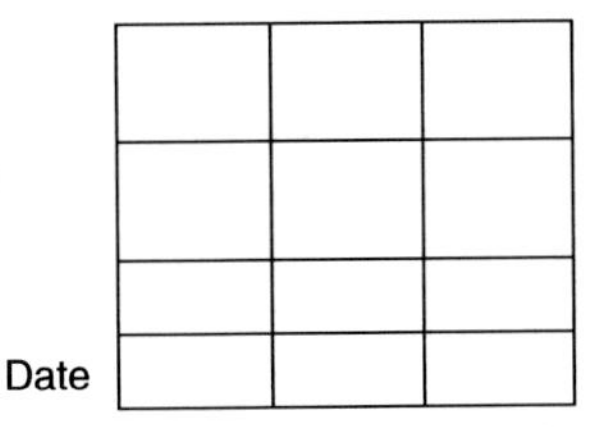

1. Affected leg flexed and foot resting, keep knee in midline. (Yes or No.)
2. From extension, flex hip in midline to more than 90° with dorsiflexed foot.
3. Return to extension maintaining dorsiflexed foot.

Date

Scale of grading

1 – some control of proximal joints

2 – as in 1, but with independent movement possible in middle joints

3 – as in 2, but with independent movement possible in distal joints

4 – good control, individual movement of distal joints but with some abnormal tonal pattern on reinforcement

5 – normal

Tone

\+ min. increased

++ mod. increased

+++ max. increased
normal

– decreased

Fig. 50 Assessment chart for stroke patients: page 2.

2. The state of muscle tone will always be assessed with great care and it must be remembered that although tonal patterns fall into two main groups, decreased and increased tone, tremor may be present and all three may coexist. 'Stovepipe' rigidity and/or clonus may be present (e.g. corpus striatum involvement, where rolling must be re-established if rehabilitation is to make any progress).

3. Previous and present exercise tolerance must be taken into account. This means that the physician–therapist relationship must be good with full communication taking place and, where necessary, GP and family help is also sought. All relevant details should be added to the final blank sheet at the end of the assessment chart.

4. The patient's outlook must be hopeful. If it is hopeless, the first requirement for successful rehabilitation is missing and all who deal with the patient must work towards altering his gloomy outlook. 'Make a cheerful approach'

Cortical integration and sensory interpretation; tactile and postural sensitivity
(Tested with eyes covered.)

Date								
Pinprick								
Joint position								
Light touch								
Two point								
Size and texture								

Grade as 'Passes', 'Failed' or 'Uncertain'

Test for hemianopia

Draw a man

Where 'Draw a man' fails, give the test '*Copy a man*'

Date			
Copy a man			
Copy a clock			
Copy a house			

Above tests to uncover neglect, agnosia and apraxia

Mental capacity

Date			
How does the patient answer simple questions?			

Any other medical history to be considered during rehabilitation?

Social background?

Any other relevant comments?

Fig. 51 Assessment chart for stroke patients: page 3.

should be added to his chart. To demonstrate progress (however little) in the early dark days almost always raises morale, and the physical approach made in this book gives early independence (again, however little) and does not defeat the patient.

5. The importance of knowing the state of the patient's vision and hearing before his stroke makes it necessary to add a note to the chart if any deficiency existed.

6. Tactile and postural sensitivity must be carefully assessed, for what must by now be very obvious reasons. For example, any loss in proprioceptive sense must be picked up in the very early days and measures taken to step up sensory input. The significance of a brief note of 'joint position' must not be overlooked and the importance of this brief note, charted as it is here, can be seen at a glance.

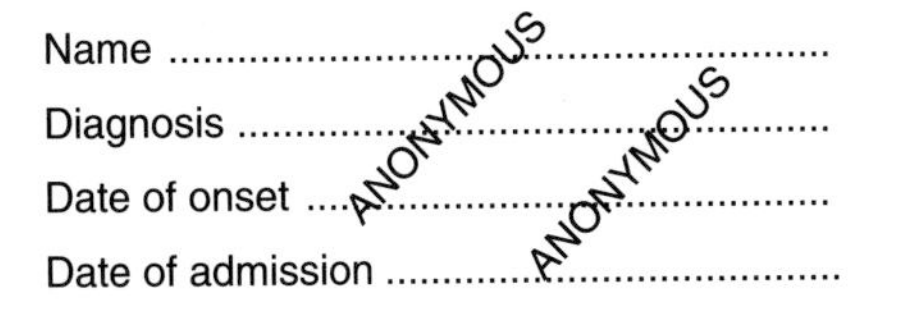
Name ....ANONYMOUS............
Diagnosis ....ANONYMOUS............
Date of onset ....
Date of admission ....

Age ......78......
Occupation ......RETIRED......
Ward ......IN-PATIENT FOR 5 MONTHS......
Date of discharge ....

Muscle tone

Are the limbs resistant to the following movements or are they heavy and abnormally relaxed?

Date	10/9/83	14/10/83	19/12/83	8/2/84	Home
Arm: movement into recovery pattern plus elevation.	F2	F1	F→S	Balanced	
Leg: movement into recovery pattern plus full flexion.	F2	F1	F→S	Balanced	

(State: resistant or heavy = spastic or flaccid = S1, 2, 3 or F1, 2, 3.)

Gross motor performance

Date	10/9/83	14/10/83	19/12/83	8/2/84	
In bed					
1. Roll from supine to right	2	3	3	3	
2. Roll from supine to left	1	3	3	3	
3. Bridging	1	3	3	3	
4. Roll to elbow propping	0	2	3	3	
5. Roll to sitting over edge of bed	0	1+	2	(2+)	
6. Sitting without use of hands	2	3	3	3	
7. Transfer from bed to chair	1	3	3	3	
In physiotherapy					
1. Rolling to prone lying	0	0	2	3	
2. Prone lying with forearm support	0	0	3	3	
3. Kneeling with forearm support	0	0	2+	3	
4. Full kneeling to stand kneeling	0	0	3	3	
5. Crawling	0	0	2	(2)	
Balance					
1. In sitting	2	3	3	3	
2. In kneeling	0	0	3	3	
3. In standing	0	0	2	(2)	

8/2/84
EXERCISES TO CONTINUE AT HOME

Weight transfers					
1. Over affected hip in sitting	0	3	3	3	
2. Over affected hand in sitting	0	2	2+	(2+)	
3. Cross R leg over L in sitting	0	0	2	3	
4. Cross L leg over R in sitting	0	0	3	3	
5. Sitting to standing with hands clasped	0	0	3	3	
6. Over affected hip in standing	0	0	2	(2)	
7. Controlled walking	0	0	1	(1+)	

SENSORY LOSS MINIMAL

Scale of grading: 3, unaided; 2, with minimal help; 1, with help; 0, impossible

Fig. 52 Partially completed page 1 of assessment chart. The red circles indicate weakness.

7. Hemianopia and visual agnosia must not be confused. This point has been fairly adequately discussed and the need for testing and charting the results of these tests will be understood.

8. Drawing tests should be carried out on separate clean sheets of paper using a felt-tipped pen. The three drawings suggested on the assessment sheet are simply there as a visual reminder for the therapist. If, for example, she wants her patient to draw a clock she presents him with a blank sheet of paper and says: 'I want you to draw a clock face with the numbers on it'. She should not stand over him (this may inhibit his performance) but she should stay near enough to watch and assess his performance. If he fails to produce any sort of coherent drawing she moves on to the copy tests. If she was testing for apraxic problems she would draw a two-dimensional house and ask him to copy it, or she might simply draw a two-dimensional diagram, e.g. a box. All drawings to be copied should be done by the therapist in front of the patient. Her drawing should be in the centre of a clean sheet of paper and then moved upwards to allow enough space to place the patient's test sheet of paper immediately below. Then she states clearly, 'Copy this box'. A space is set aside on the assessment chart for the date of the test. There is also a space on the assessment chart for a comment from the team member who conducts the test; this information is then available for the rest of the team. The comment will sum up the drawing tests. It might read: 'Neglect of left half of space' or 'Major perceptual disorder' or 'Agnosia and disturbance of body image'.

9. 'Mental capacity' might be better described as 'orientation'. Simple questions testing memory and awareness of environment are asked. This test will not be suitable for the deaf or aphasic patient. Examples of questions asked are:

- 'What is your name?'
- 'What is your address?'
- 'What day is it?'
- 'What month is it?'
- 'What year is it?'
- 'What time is it?' (The patient is allowed to consult his watch or a clock or to give the time to the nearest hour.)
- 'What hospital is this?'
- 'How long have you been here?'
- 'What is your date of birth?'

Recent memory may be easily and simply tested by the therapist. For example she may remove the patient's shoes for an exercise session and say to him: 'Look, I am putting your shoes in the cupboard'. Ten minutes later she will ask: 'Where are your shoes?'.

ASSESSING THE APHASIC PATIENT

Many of the suggested tests are not suitable for the aphasic patient. The definition of aphasia is an inability to express thought in words; loss of the faculty of interchanging thought, with the intellect or will remaining unaffected. Bearing in mind Sandra Jackson Anderson's comments above regarding dysphasia, one can only reiterate the urgent need to include a skilled speech therapist in any assessment of the patient with a breakdown in communication, or with any suspected problems that come within the speech therapist's area. Where there is a shortage of such therapists, this need may be met by having just one such therapist who is not a resident member of a complete working unit, but who may be called in to make the necessary assessment in the hospital or home situation.

If expert follow-up treatments are judged to be necessary the shortage of skilled speech therapists can still cause problems. In such a situation it can be helpful if the speech therapist can pass on suggestions to the stroke team about what to do, and what not to do.

THE IMPORTANCE OF RECORDING PROGRESS

Whatever the method chosen to record assessment findings and to plan a treatment programme, careful records should be kept and treatment progress noted. Set realistic goals and adjust the programme to meet any changing situation. Much will depend on the therapist's cheerful approach and the rapport established between the patient and his helpers (therapists, doctors, nurses and family members).

ONE MORE PROBLEM

Before leaving this section on assessment and problems to be addressed, there is one more difficulty that has to be mentioned. It has been left until last, not because it is unimportant, but rather because it is of great importance to any patient who is afflicted in this way, and is placed here as a reminder that it should not be overlooked: the problem of bowel trouble.

This is a fairly common problem after stroke. Unfortunately it is frequently misunderstood and misinterpreted. It may present as constipation or diarrhoea but, where diarrhoea is a persistent complication, it must always be remembered that this can be (and with stroke patients frequently is) a complication of constipation. It results from leakage past an impacted faecal mass. Loss of tone, inactivity where the patient formerly led an active life and an unsuitable diet for controlling the consequent bowel failure are all contributory factors.

Formerly, this condition was common among children suffering from poliomyelitis, and routine manual evacuation of the bowels was standard procedure. I see no reason to suppose that, as in the patient suffering from poliomyelitis, the patient suffering from a stroke should not be expected to have similar problems. I have myself come across this problem in very many stroke victims and I feel very strongly that it is one aspect of treatment that is often sadly neglected.

All members of the team should be aware of bowel disorder and its consequences, as it can have such an adverse effect on rehabilitation. The patient suffering from constipation feels out of sorts and thoroughly depressed and the effectiveness of his stroke rehabilitation is considerably reduced, if not halted. I would go so far as to say that in some cases the effectiveness of treatment is so badly impaired that there is a reverse into steady physical deterioration. Constipation is a very common underlying cause of depression.

A final thought or question: surely the use of an indwelling catheter is not the way to retrain a weak bladder after a stroke?

REFERENCES

Eggers O 1983 Occupational therapy in the treatment of adult hemiplegia. Heinemann, London

Jackson Anderson S 1987 In: Johnstone M Home care for the stroke patient, 2nd edn. Churchill Livingstone, Edinburgh

Johnstone M 1989 Thirty-five single-patient case study on an elderly population. Physiotherapy 75: 7

7

CONCLUSIONS, REVISION AND UPDATE

GENERAL COMMENTS

The sensorimotor approach to stroke rehabilitation as presented here is a reasoned and satisfying approach which gives consistently good results. With a breakdown in the finely balanced facilitatory–inhibitory principle on which the neuromuscular system depends, all who care for the stroke patient (nurses or therapists) should act as extended facilitatory–inhibitory agents until normal responses are re-established and cortical control regained.

Using the method described in this book, this is what is done. All involved work to:

1. inhibit dominant reflexes which follow dominant antigravity patterns
2. facilitate lost responses and normal reflexes
3. step up sensory input
4. re-establish all lost responses
5. facilitate effective cortical control and feedback.

Statistics tell us that:

1. a stroke is the third commonest cause of admission to hospital
2. there is an early mortality rate
3. the survivors have a relatively good prognosis

but

4. there is an ever-increasing reservoir of stroke survivors waiting for rehabilitation.

We have not done well enough in the past. There is much work to be done. Recovery from a stroke involves a way of life. It is similar to going on a slimming diet, in that it is not a way of life that is followed for a few days, or spasmodically, but one that will continue without interruption for many weeks until recovery has fulfilled the individual's maximum recovery potential.

Sometimes recovery slows down and rests for a little while. It is a mistake to say at this stage that recovery has plateaued! Refuse to give up easily. It is a way of life that is built round basic positioning, much of which the patient can be taught to undertake by himself.

Not surprisingly, to initiate a family member into the best way to handle and care for the stroke victim would seem to be essential. If possible, welcome a family member into the team approach early after the onset of the stroke. Do not think this is too much to ask of families, or that it would place too great a demand on one person. Nowadays many stroke patients have to be cared for in the home environment and to follow the method suggested here will quite quickly lead to easy handling and a fair degree of independence for the patient.

LOCATION OF THE PATIENT'S FURNITURE

Start with the nurse or with the person who carries out the nursing duties.

First get the location of the patient's furniture into therapeutic order. Figure 53 shows the correct location of the patient's furniture. Figure 53A does not indicate the patient's positioning; it just shows which is his disabled side. Note that the chair in Figure 53B is placed very close to the bed. Training always in the same way will lead to independence. This is one situation in which the patient is allowed to support himself with his sound side by leaning on the bed as he transfers to the chair. In the home situation, when safe independent transfer from bed to chair is well established, this next transfer becomes possible (Fig. 53C). Note that the commode must not be on wheels.

Figure 54 illustrates a suitable chair and table used to maintain inhibiting positions. The chair should be the correct height for the patient to sit with knees and ankles flexed to 90°, heels resting on the floor. The patient with short legs usually needs a footstool for positioning purposes. The table should be the correct height to allow for forearm leaning, with the hemiplegic arm parallel with the red stripe, and weight must be transmitted firmly from elbow to shoulder. As quickly as possible the patient should be taught that his hand must not stray across the red stripe. Provided the shoulder position is in the correct inhibiting pattern, this is also a good situation in which to use the half-arm splint, or, with pillow support (the pillow held in place by the arm of the chair and the table) the long arm splint can be put to good use. Do not over-inflate these splints and always check that the patient's fingertips are well back inside the splint. (See also point 6 in the section on extensor spasticity in the leg, p. 111).

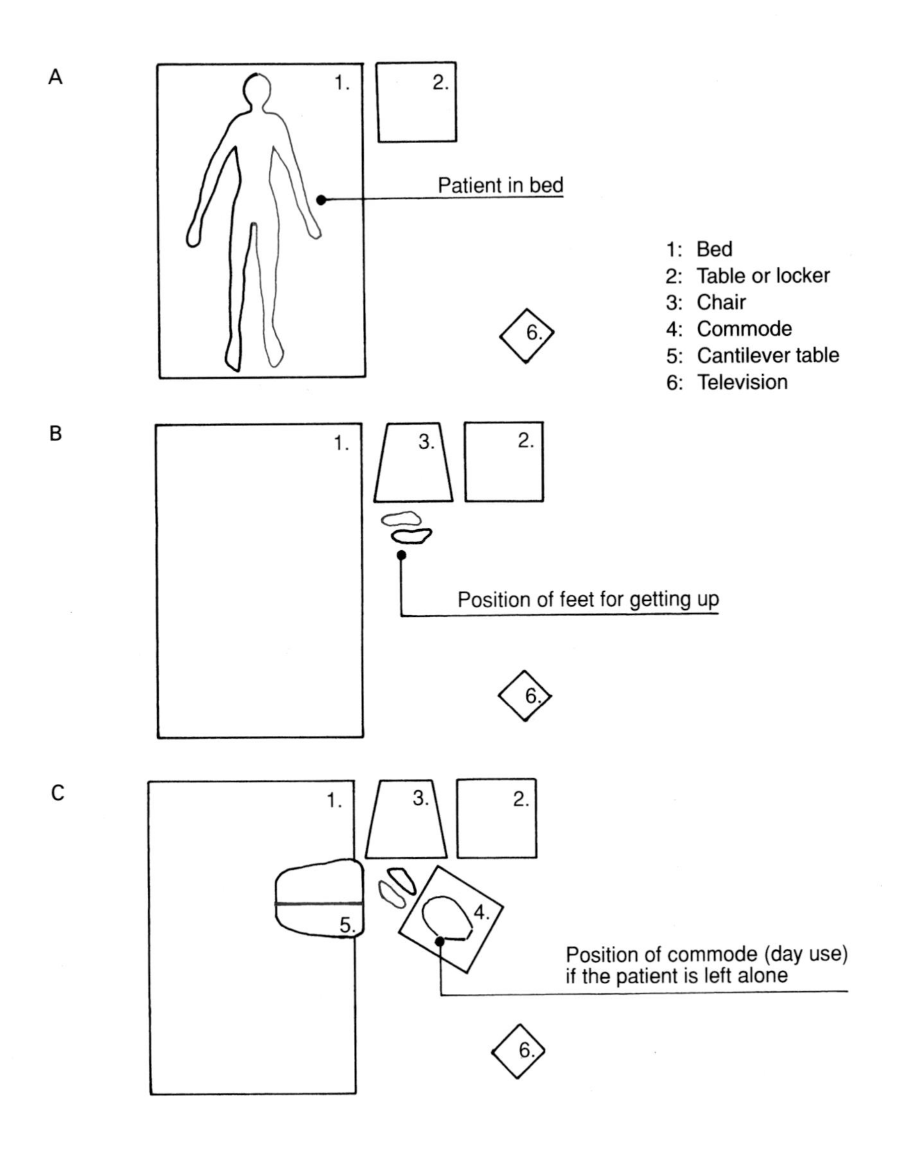

Fig. 53 Location of patient's furniture for use in the home. Note that for night use the commode must be placed in position 3 (the chair's position beside the bed).

SUMMARY OF THE TREATMENT CONCEPT

The tenets of the rehabilitation concept are summarized here.

1. Voluntary muscles, even when at rest, are always maintained in a state of mild contraction which is called muscle tone and which is more marked in the muscles which hold the body upright against gravity.

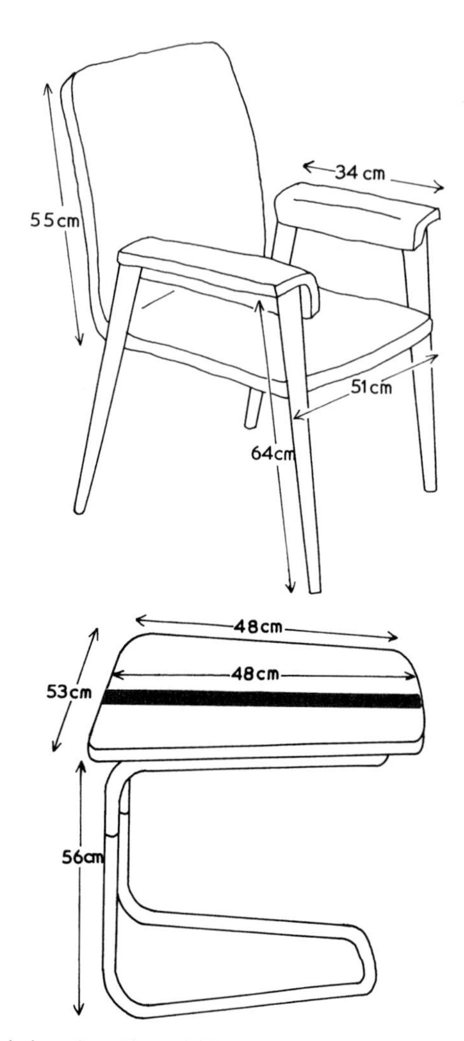

Fig. 54 A suitable chair and cantilever table.

2. The structures responsible for the maintenance of normal muscle tone are the cerebral cortex or higher cerebral region, the vestibular system and spinal cord, the muscle spindles, Golgi tendon organs and the anterior horn cells.
3. Muscle tone is entirely reflex in character and is directly based on the spinal reflex arc.
4. Where normal muscle tone is missing there can be no normal controlled movement.
5. The vital missing function that faces stroke patients is loss of normal muscle tone on the affected side. The stroke patient is faced with developing spasticity, movement loss and usually some degree of sensory loss. Even where there is a severe degree of hypotonus present, with the passage of time, a developing hypertonus will be found in the antigravity muscles, first noticed creeping into the fingers.

6. To re-establish normal movement it is necessary to re-establish normal muscle tone. We base our rehabilitation programme on redevelopment of controlled movement in response to reflex activity.

7. All true stroke rehabilitation must begin at spinal reflex level and work upwards to cortical level. This means beginning at spinal reflex level and working upward to midbrain responses, using tonic neck reflexes and labyrinthine reflexes, until basal responses are gained, bringing in righting reflexes and equilibrium responses. Basal responses must be established before cortical level can be effective.

8. To follow an effective rehabilitation programme as described in point 7 above, the physiotherapist sets out to restore controlled movement following the pattern demonstrated in the motor development of the infant. This motor development pattern, when applied to stroke rehabilitation, is most easily understood and most effective if it is seen and practised as two distinct routines: (a) rolling to sitting to standing to walking; (b) rolling to prone to propping on forearms to crawling to kneeling to standing to walking.

9. The aim is to get back to cortical level so that dominant reflexes are once more integrated into cortical control.

10. The pattern of spasticity bears a direct relationship to the dominating reflexes.

11. The physiotherapist, and all those who handle stroke patients, must act as the inhibiting influence on hypertonic motor neurones until the missing postural reflex mechanism is re-established, and normal inhibiting influences restored. This is done by making sure that the stroke patient is maintained in the antispasticity (or recovery) pattern 24 hours a day and that rehabilitation is carried out within this pattern. In other words, correct positioning is used as an inhibiting influence on hyperactive motor neurones (or developing spasticity) until inhibition from cortical level is re-established and normal muscle tone restored.

12. All movements of the affected limbs will be passive, assisted and active assisted movements (working through these progressive stages), the operator maintaining the initiative and preventing the release of dominant reflex activity, until static reflexes are once more integrated into controlled movement.

13. Side-lying positions, which do not increase extensor tone, will be used wherever possible. Therefore, where it is necessary to increase extensor tone in the arm using the supine position and neck extension, the legs will be positioned with extra care. Where it is necessary to leave the patient in supine lying for any length of time, the legs must be positioned with great care and the head will not be supported by raised pillows to give neck flexion.

14. If early shoulder elevation with external rotation gives pain it is reasonable to assume that the patient is not being nursed and handled with due care and correct positioning is not being maintained. Also, correct movement patterns may not have been established.

15. To teach the patient to compensate with his sound side is a disservice. For example, to teach him to hook his sound foot under his affected foot to assist the movement of his affected leg when getting out of bed, is to teach him a habit which will ruin the correct sequence of development of controlled movement (destroying the rolling pattern) and will later pose very difficult problems.

16. Treatment must begin early after the onset of the stroke and must be intensive and repetitive if the best possible results are to be obtained.

17. Positioning in the spasticity pattern, working into the spasticity pattern, allowing drift into the spasticity pattern, making excessive demands, and encouraging early, willed, voluntary effort, will all serve to stimulate unwanted dominant reflex activity and must be discarded from any treatment plan. This also means that the patient will not be asked to lead an activity with an area of disability until muscle tone is restored to normal. For example, he should not be allowed to use his hand in any way without forearm support until he can place his arm in space from any position and hold it there in the full recovery pattern (start with the trunk and maintain arm stability with the inflatable splint).

18. If the spinal reflex arc (which maintains normal muscle tone) is disrupted by lesion of the motor nerves, the sensory nerves or the reflex centres, normal muscle tone will be lost. This is because the ventral (or anterior) horn of grey matter in the spinal cord contains vital cells which receive impulses from the proprioceptors along sensory neurones and from the motor area of the cerebral cortex.

19. All movement is a direct response to sensory stimuli from vision, hearing, superficial pressure and deep pressure.

20. If demand (or sensory stimulation) from the higher centres of the brain is missing or impaired, it must be stepped up by adding stimuli from the proprioceptors, and, with increased demand, a response will be gained.

21. With missing or impaired postural or proprioceptive sense, sensory input must be stepped up dramatically if there is to be any hope of re-establishing the postural reflex mechanism. Proprioceptors must be bombarded with stimuli until the ventral horn is activated or a response is gained.

22. To stimulate antigravity and postural mechanisms use intensive rolling, weightbearing and all pressure techniques.

23. Where severe handicap is present because the servo system concerned in antigravity and postural mechanisms lacks proprioception, the pressure splint, using both intermittent and sustained pressure, has supplied the necessary force to bridge the gap in a large number of cases.

24. Where the dominating reflexes are removed from normal inhibiting influences, the pressure splint, in this case with sustained pressure and so inflated orally to make the inner sleeve mould to the arm, acts as a most effective inhibiting influence if it is correctly applied.

25. In all cases, weightbearing through the affected limbs in the inhibiting pattern is vital to recovery. This means gravity approximation; gravity approximation increased by manual pressure, and full weightbearing. All these should take place through a correctly positioned base, and remembering that weightbearing through the heel of the hand is as important as that through the heel of the foot. Weightbearing in an uninhibited pattern will step up spasticity.

26. The final sequence of distal-to-proximal movement re-education must be undertaken to reach a satisfactory standard of rehabilitation. Unless the stroke patient is able to stand on his affected hand, i.e. put full weight through his hand as in crawling, he will not free the primitive flexor grasp and develop controlled hand movements.

27. In the stroke patient, with a breakdown in the finely balanced facilitatory–inhibitory mechanism on which the neuromuscular system depends, the physiotherapist must act as an extended facilitatory–inhibitory agent, until normal responses are re-established and cortical control regained. With the introduction of pressure splints to maintain inhibiting limb patterns, there is also much that occupational therapists can add to the recovery programme. With all other team members taking part in the essential use of inhibiting positioning, the stroke patient has a better prospect of physical recovery than ever before.

28. Early weightbearing in inhibiting patterns is essential, e.g. weightbearing through the forearm with a suitable forearm support (see Fig. 17). The patient, wherever possible, ought to begin correct weightbearing within 2 or 3 days after the onset of the stroke; otherwise, it will later be found that his brain has accepted wrong movement patterns and he will not readily transfer his weight over to his affected side. Where he has been taught to do this with skilled supporting help in the very early days, many of the otherwise very difficult problems of stroke rehabilitation do not even occur. This must include correct weightbearing compression on both limbs, arm and leg, and correct weightbearing support in sitting and lying positions 24 hours a day. Never forget the special needs of the stroke shoulder.

29. The arm is mobilized into outward rotation; the leg is mobilized into inward rotation.

30. No amount of treatment will result in the patient's full potential for recovery if spasticity is not attacked 24 hours a day.

THE USE OF THE PRESSURE SPLINT: A SUMMARY

The pressure splint is an effective aid towards skilled rehabilitation of the affected arm in stroke care. Using a carefully planned pressure splint procedure, which must include a series of progressive exercises, the splint works as a most effective treatment aid for the following reasons:

1. It inhibits unwanted excessive antigravity tone, when it is correctly applied, so that it holds the arm in the full antispasticity pattern.

2. Muscle tone may be influenced by pressure on the fingertips from the splint, the fingertips being a key point of control from which the strength and distribution of muscle tone in the rest of the body may be influenced.

3. Relaxation of the arm occurs when the Golgi organs are stimulated by contracting muscles pulling on their tendons, prolonged static contraction leading to relaxation. Where the splint is properly applied the prolonged static stretch is made possible. Golgi organs are the specialized sensory receptors, or proprioceptors, in the musculotendinous junction and are receptive to stretch. Unlike other proprioceptors, or the stretch receptors of muscle spindles, Golgi organs are known to have an inhibitory effect upon motoneurone pools of their own muscle supply – an autogenic, i.e. self-generating, effect.

4. Sensory input is stepped up by the careful and efficient use of the splint, e.g. as in weightbearing techniques.

5. The stability of sustained posture necessary for effective advancing exercise techniques is supplied by the splint.

6. Associated reactions, which always follow dominant tonal patterns, are controlled by the splint and tonal overflow is directed into the nondominant low tonal pattern.

7. A rigid splint should never be used. Muscles will contract against such a splint and increase the disability. The inflatable splint depends on all over even pressure. Without the stability and control of muscle tone offered by the inflatable pressure splint, the motor development rehabilitation programme presented in this book would not be possible, particularly where full recovery of the hemiplegic arm is concerned. Recovery of the arm with a return to skilled function is an outcome devoutly to be sought and of supreme importance to the stroke victim. Therapy professions involved in stroke rehabilitation cannot afford to ignore this valuable aid towards recovery.

For the above seven reasons, use of the pressure splint in the re-education of normal function in an arm that has been affected by a stroke makes sound sense. Prolonged stretch of ½–1 hour is often found to be most effective with an immediate reduction of spasticity in the shoulder which can be felt manually by the therapist. She should then follow this with upper trunk and shoulder mobilizing while maintaining inhibiting patterns (the splint still in place).

As soon as practicable, exercise for the arm must include weight bearing from the heel of the hand through an extended elbow to an outwardly rotated shoulder. The pressure splint makes this possible from an early date.

Intermittent pressure has been found to have a place in treatment where proprioceptive sense is diminished. When used, techniques using sustained pressure must also be included in treatment sessions.

Contraindications to intermittent pressure. It should not be used on patients with acute pulmonary oedema, and should be used with caution on those where pre-existing deep vein thrombosis is suspected. In conditions where an anticoagulant has been prescribed and blood tests have shown the prothrombin level to be stabilized, e.g. stroke patients who had rheumatic fever in their younger days, intermittent pressure may be used.

A RECENT DEVELOPMENT IN PRESSURE SPLINTS

Double chamber arm splints in all three lengths can now be obtained:

1. long arm splint, length 80 cm, two chambers
2. long arm splint, length 70 cm, two chambers
3. half-arm splint, length 51 cm, two chambers.

METHOD OF APPLICATION

This is exactly as given for the single chamber splint but inflate the posterior chamber first to gain an extensor response into the full extension pattern of recovery. Inflate firmly to hold this inhibitory pattern. Next put a little air into the anterior chamber to stabilize and give a cushioned comfort. Finally, check that the posterior section has not been overinflated.

Warning. It is all too easy to overinflate this splint. The pressure which is added to the anterior section will increase the posterior pressure. Therefore always check the posterior pressure before you leave your patient.

These splints are not to be used to replace the single chamber splints. A number of therapists have asked for two chamber splints and these can have a place where spasticity presents problems.

For application, position the patient as in Figure 7 but with both knees bent up as in the bridging position, with pillow support if necessary. Inflate the splint as in Figure 23B, but inflate the posterior chamber first. Should a mistake be made and the anterior chamber be inflated first over the palm of the hand a resulting flexor response would be stimulated. After a firm inflation has been given to the posterior chamber, followed by a lesser inflation to the anterior chamber, check that the pressure in the posterior chamber is not excessive.

Before inflating the splint impress on your patient that he must lie very still and must not lift his head because this would increase the spasticity in his arm. A greater input to the inhibitory arm pattern is given if his head is maintained with mild neck extension (as in Fig. 7) but also combine this with head rotation to the affected side. With the two chamber splint in place as described, it makes sound sense to give the patient a rest period of ½–1 hour before starting the exercise session.

AN AID TO STROKE REHABILITATION: THE ROCKING CHAIR

A rocking chair is an invaluable aid in all stroke rehabilitation. The patient makes use of the almost spontaneous movement that results from sitting in the chair, particularly where music with a marked rhythm is played. It is usually necessary to give the patient a firm footstool to raise the level of his feet so that his knees are flexed to 90°, and he will push on his heels to rock the chair.

Following the introduction of the rocking chair, and a lengthy period of observation in the clinical setting, it was seen that rehabilitation was given a dynamic boost and a good walking gait was more easily achieved; but, as sitting is the position of greatest flexor tone in the forearm with a consequent build-up of spasticity, I used the URIAS orally inflated full arm splint to inhibit this unwanted antigravity tone in the elbow, wrist and fingers while the patient rocked in the chair.

However, I felt that it ought to be possible to give the hemiplegic arm a more dynamic treatment. I saw a need for a firm weight-bearing base to support the splinted arm so that each rock of the chair would give a useful thrust from the heel of the hand through an extended elbow to an outwardly rotated shoulder. In other words, the patient would be using his arm in the inhibiting pattern giving a repetitive thrust through the positioned hand with each rock

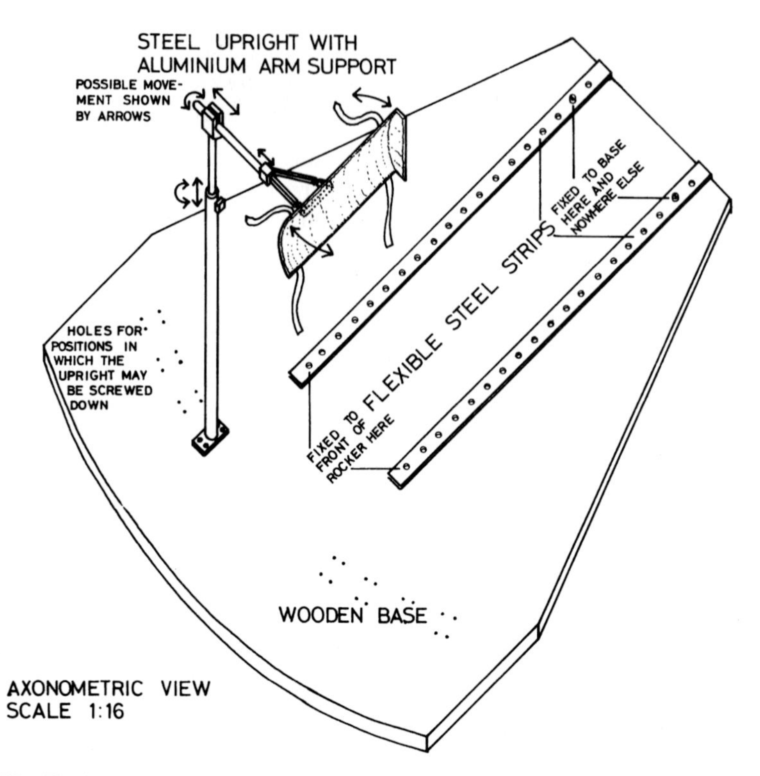

Fig. 55 The base of the Law rocking machine.

of the chair. I sought the help of bioengineer Dr H T Law of Edinburgh University and the result of our collaboration is illustrated in Figures 55 and 56.

Figure 55 is a draughtsman's drawing of the apparatus base and upright for the hand support (i.e. the apparatus minus the chair).

Figure 56 shows a patient using the apparatus. Dr Law had solved the problem of allowing the chair to rock without moving its position and he had provided a fixed base to support the hand while maintaining the inhibiting pattern of the arm. The height and rotation of the upright (see Fig. 55), and the length and rotation of the horizontal arm and angle of the hand rest were all adjustable to suit the individual patient. The URIAS splint must be carefully applied and inflated by mouth before positioning the patient's arm in the apparatus. A firm pad should be added to give supporting pressure behind the scapula as illustrated. Flexible steel strips had been fastened to the front of both rockers and to the back of the chipboard base and nowhere else. This gives the chair its ability to rock on a fixed base.

After 2 years of testing this apparatus in the clinical field, I decided it had much to offer towards rehabilitation of the hemiplegic shoulder and arm. However, this should not be surprising. It fulfils already accepted principles of rehabilitation in this specialized field. Techniques aimed at producing upper trunk rotation and shoulder stability received dynamic treatment, as

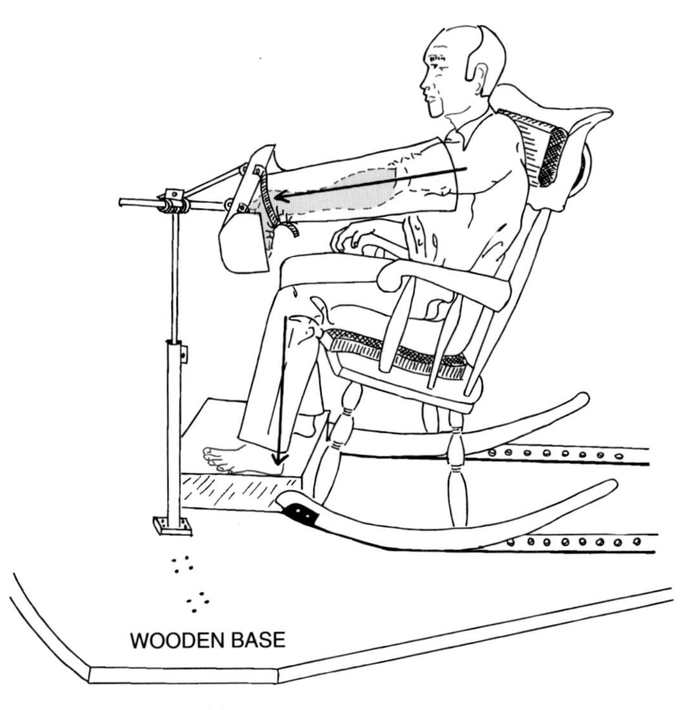

Fig. 56 The Law rocking machine.

did sensory loss, and it seemed that arm recovery gained a significant and very satisfactory boost which should not be ignored. I have kept careful progress notes illustrated by photographs to give a visual aid to progress assessment. I have tested patients with severe flaccidity or extreme spasticity several weeks or months after the onset of a stroke. Results have shown impressive improvement. I have been surprised most by the progress it is possible to make with the flaccid limb with severe sensory loss. Two years is not a long clinical trial, but, where possible this trial continues, and 2 years with access to a fair number of patients convinced me that we had succeeded in producing a piece of apparatus that should not be ignored. It maintains the inhibiting position for the whole of the hemiplegic side of the body and, provided the rocking of the chair comes from heel pressure as shown in Figure 56, it gives a repetitive therapeutic exercise which adheres to our recovery criteria. I have since seen it in use in Switzerland, Belgium, Portugal, England and America. Using Scottish country dance music gives an obvious boost to motivation.

NEUROPLASTICITY

The subject of neuroplasticity should be mentioned in any update on treatment.

Up-to-date neurological teaching has now advanced into the realm of neuroplasticity. When I attended one of Professor Kidd's early teaching sessions on this subject, I first became aware of the exciting advances that the researchers in neurology were making and I began to understand what was meant by the term 'neuroplasticity'. Since then, as far as I have been able, I have followed this up-to-date teaching and it seems to me that the review of neuroplasticity presented by Richard Stephenson (1993), is well worth careful study. So, how does this affect the method of stroke rehabilitation as presented in this book? In my mind it is all very encouraging and adds to the credibility of the rehabilitation method presented here.

In Chapter 1 of this book I have quoted a sentence from Richard Stephenson's review because it so clearly presented a treatment principle proven to be true through many years of practice in the clinical field.

> *Latent areas of the brain can specialise to replace lost function and new pathways can form to by-pass the effects of lesions.*

Stephenson also states:

> *However, to achieve this successfully, intensive, repeated stimulation is required to place demands on the reorganising systems.*

As already stated, constant repetition of the exercises in the advancing rehabilitation programme is required; a constant demand to gain a response. However, this will only be successful if the exercises use and maintain inhibiting patterns and increase sensory input. To do this is to establish a sound foundation which allows the reorganizing systems of the brain to replace lost function.

Treatment results have already confirmed my commitment to the method of rehabilitation presented in this book, but, the more I learn about neuroplasticity, the more I understand that here indeed is neurological confirmation of my rehabilitation approach. The former, commonly held belief that neuronal connections once formed are fixed and unchanging is no longer accepted. Once again developmental patterns come to mind. As the infant develops into an adult, new nerve connections are made over many years. The question to be asked and answered concerns this continuing reorganization of connections: does this take place after the brain damage of stroke?

From the point of view of the rehabilitation of lost function resulting from the brain damage of stroke, the fact that 'latent areas of the brain can specialise to replace lost function' is probably the single most important fact to emerge from recent research. My understanding of this research is that it gives one more important reason for following the infant's developmental patterns, with constant repetition to assist in reordering of connections in the brain, opening up new pathways and restoring lost skills; a constant demand to gain a response. There is plasticity in the central nervous system. Present a rehabilitation situation which makes full use of this fact and give it time to happen.

Once again I am indebted to the Open University for the excellent course *Brain, Biology and Behaviour*, this time for the teaching on plasticity in the central nervous system. This section was presented by Sean Murphy and speakers from the National Institute for Medical Research (Dr Geoff Raceman and Dr Tim Bliss) and University College London (Professor Pat Wall), all presenting their involvement in research (Murphy et al 1980). Sean Murphy presented their findings under the headings of 'Development', 'Recovery' and 'Learning', each having a bearing on reordering of connections in the brain.

1. Development: there is persistent development of new axons and formation of new synapses as shown by Dr Geoff Raceman.
2. Recovery: synapses which were silent or inactive can become active and respond to the nearest latent area, as illustrated by Professor Pat Wall.
3. Learning: the efficiency of existing synapses is capable of being enhanced, as presented by Dr Tim Bliss.

In any one area of the nervous system all of these could form the basis for recovery of function after damage.

After a stroke has affected the brain neurosensory cells continue growing. Recovery of the postural reflex mechanism is vital, and rehabilitation measures must be taken at once, to make it possible for physical recovery of muscles and movement to begin before altered muscle tone, sensory loss plus loss of the memory of normal movement have taken over, leaving the unfortunate stroke victim helpless in the face of ever-increasing disability. The rehabilitation measures to be taken have been carefully set out in this book; but the good news presented to us by research neurologists is that after a stroke neurosensory cells continue growing. Where one area is knocked out, the neurosensory cells respond to the nearest new area, synapses remain which were silent but are now altered in the new area, and open up new pathways. However, this takes time. As sound rehabilitation practice continues, the new cells send axons into the brain, replacing lost function, and the development of lost skills takes place.

My interpretation of this teaching is that it underlines the urgency of the need to establish a sound rehabilitation programme in the very early days of treatment. Each patient ought to be given the chance of fulfilling his maximum recovery potential. For example, where proprioception is deficient, sensory input to the brain is deficient. With deficient input, appropriate output will be deficient. Rehabilitation must address this problem by using techniques which bombard and stimulate proprioceptors. The recovering brain needs this dynamic boost to sensory input. 'The efficiency of existing synapses is capable of being enhanced.' It would seem logical to suggest that the sensorimotor approach as described here, which has given consistently satisfactory results, lays down a sound foundation with an increasing demand which allows the reorganizing systems of the brain to replace lost function.

A word of warning: when it comes to recovery of lost skills, do not increase the demand before the patient has reached the required recovery level. For example, work with keyboards and all the skills of modern computing should not be pushed at the patient early in the recovery programme. This may seem like an extreme example but I have seen it happen! The result of sitting a patient at a keyboard too soon after the onset of his brain damage will lead to awful frustration, an all too rapid build-up of spasticity, and the deep depression that comes with his realization of his own inadequacy. Give the damaged brain time to set about the reorganizing process; give neuroplasticity a chance.

POSITIONING (Figs 57–60)

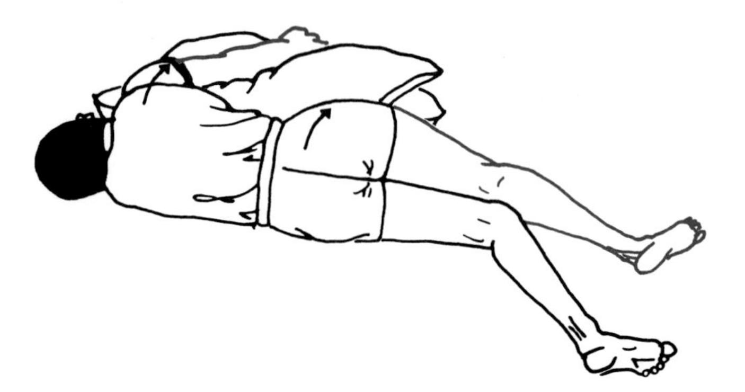

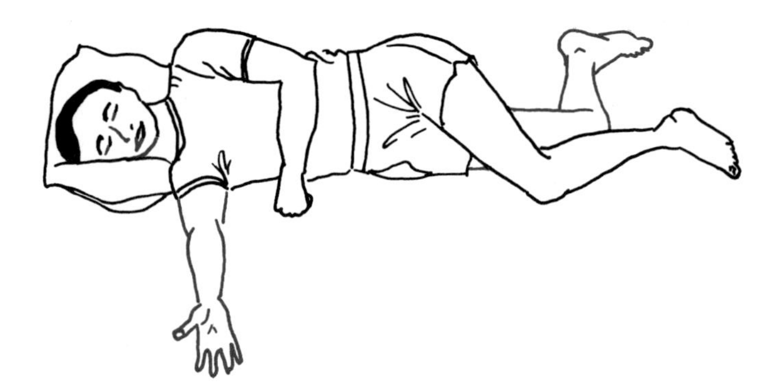

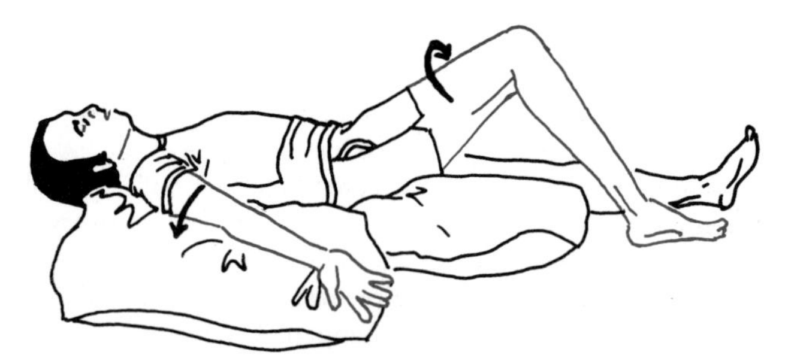

Fig. 57 Revision of positioning: right-sided disability.

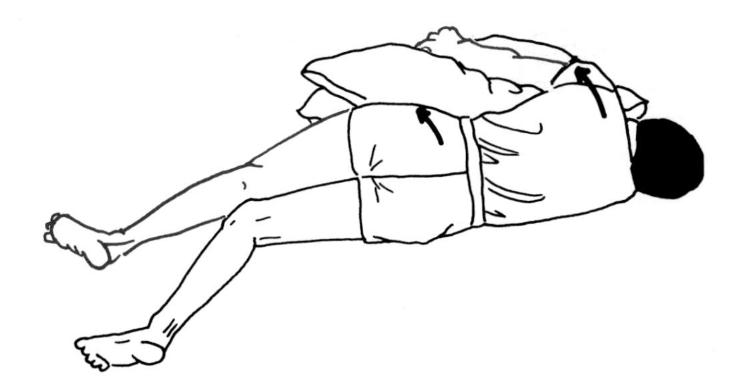

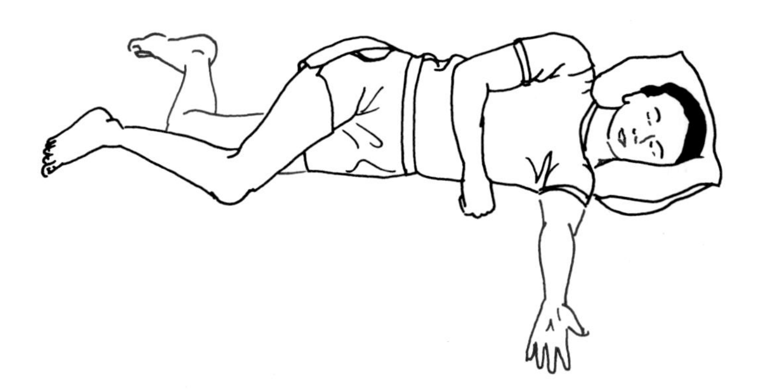

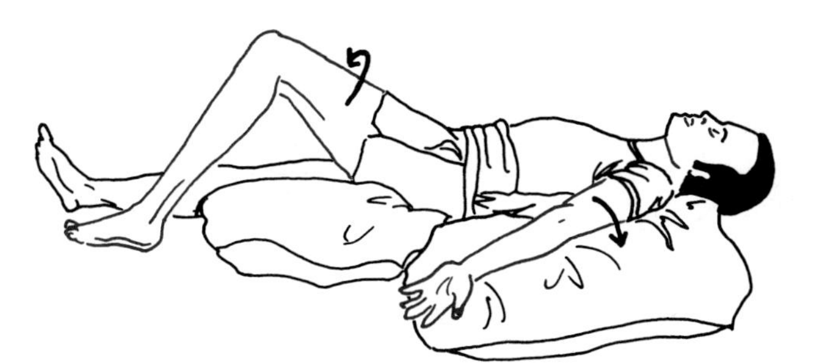

Fig. 58 Revision of positioning: left-sided disability.

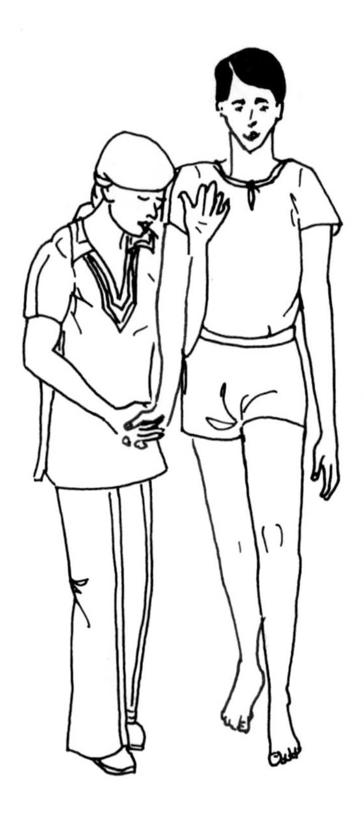

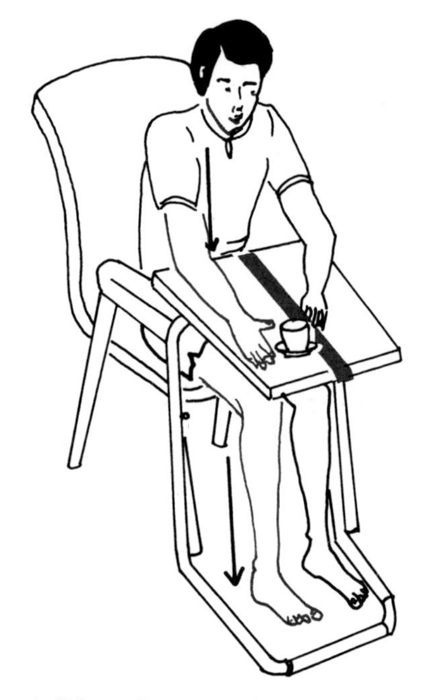

Fig. 59 Maintain inhibiting positioning at all times. It very soon becomes a way of life.

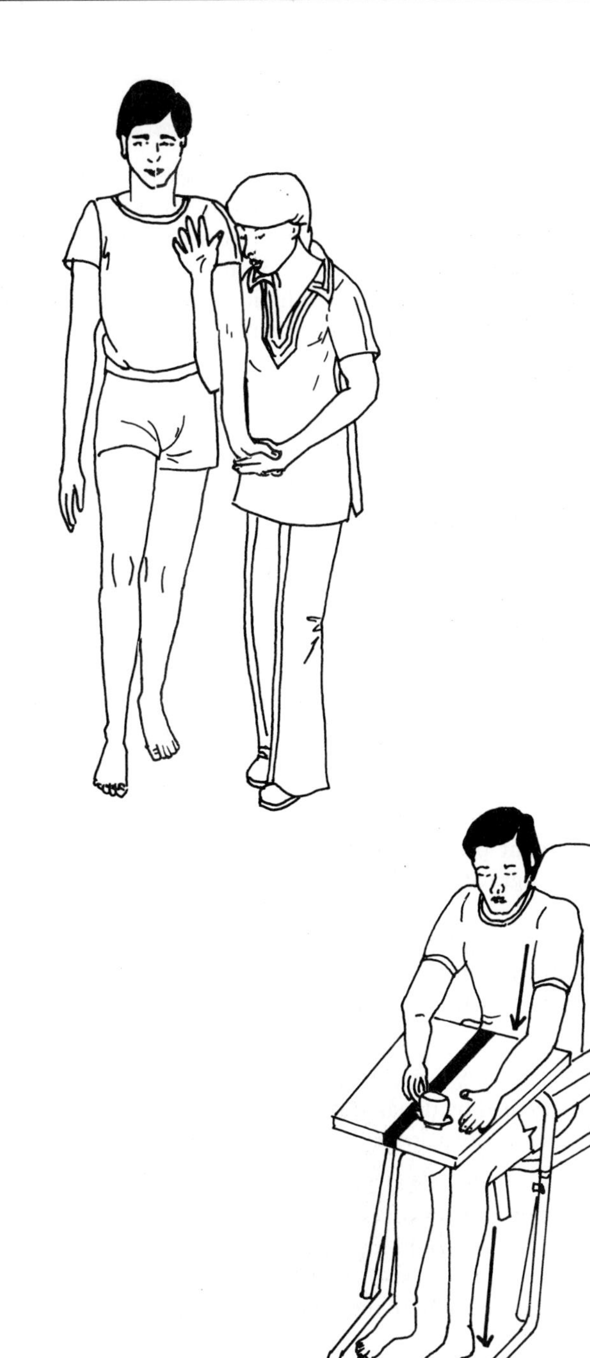

Fig. 60 Always handle the patient on his disabled side.

FINAL THOUGHTS (WITH SOME REPETITION!)

The sensorimotor approach to stroke rehabilitation as described here is a reasoned and satisfying approach which gives consistently good results. With the breakdown in the finely balanced facilitatory–inhibitory principle on which the neuromuscular system depends, therapists and all who care for stroke patients must act as an extended facilitatory–inhibitory agent until normal responses are re-established and cortical control regained.

1. Abnormal muscle tone must be taken into account.
2. There is almost always a need to restore normal sensation.

This means that reciprocal innervation must be restored; that is that the missing inhibition which controls the stretch reflex, allowing smooth action to take place between antagonistic pairs of muscles, must be replaced by mechanical means (inhibitory positioning and inhibitory patterns of movement) to be used at all times while rehabilitation is undertaken and, at the same time, sensory input must be dynamic.

This means that all therapists should be aware of the total tonal patterns that will occur with all movement and, in particular, of the alteration that will occur in the hemiplegic side of the patient's body with every movement made with his sound side, because of reflex activity. For example: never give the patient a walking stick to use on his sound side. To do this is to destroy the rehabilitation progress. He will simply learn to lean on the stick and to substitute lost function in his affected side by compensating with his sound side. From then on treatment progress will stop because he is now steadily producing non-inhibited antigravity tonal patterns (associated reactions) on his affected side.

Integrating inflatable pressure splints into the rehabilitation programme will supply the missing limb stability using the inhibitory pattern and, at the same time, increase sensory input, which is greatly enhanced by:

1. pressure from the splint
2. early stability which makes early weightbearing possible
3. intermittent pressure supplied by the altering pressures (e.g. weight transfers) during exercise sessions and by the use of a mechanical pump.

Do not overinflate the splint. If the initial pressure given feels very hard when the operator grasps the splint and squeezes it, then let a little air out to give a slight spongy feel. Never go above 40 mmHg. It is helpful, when students are taught to do this, to have them test the pressure with the gauge from a sphygmomanometer until they are able to make an accurate test by hand.

REFERENCES

Stephenson R 1993 A review of neuroplasticity. Physiotherapy 79: 10
Murphy S, Raceman G, Bliss T, Wall P 1980 Biology, brain and behaviour. Plasticity in the central nervous system. Open University course

CASE HISTORY 1

A case history is presented here to illustrate the effects of integrating pressure splints and pressure techniques into a rehabilitation programme after a stroke.

As has already been emphasized, rehabilitation should start as early as possible after the onset of a stroke, giving severe deformities no time to develop. The patient illustrated in the following photographs underwent late treatment; late, that is, with the introduction of pressure splint techniques. She had been treated with what is so often regarded as a reasonably sound approach to rehabilitation and had been considered able to return to live at home but, 2 years after the stroke, she presented with quite severe problems.

1. Marked left-sided spasticity.
2. Reduced sensation.
3. Compensating with her right side.
4. Walking with the support of a stick in her right hand.
5. Walking with circumduction and hip retraction of the left leg, the leg being little more than a prop.
6. Inverted spasticity of the left foot which was painful, and she constantly tripped over the toes making walking dangerous.
7. Postural stability had not been obtained; transference of weight to the affected side of her body was poor.
8. Her fear of open space was very obvious. Because of this she was unwilling to be left in the house alone but frightened to go out of the house, even with her husband supporting her on her sound side. This was one of the first things to be changed: he had to learn to support her on her affected side! His visits to the golf course were no longer possible.
9. On the plus side he put a brave face on his lack of golf but he longed to have at least a game a week. This was an important point to note in his assessment. It is important to make a thorough assessment of home back-up.
10. Again on the plus side, she herself was positively motivated with a strong desire to improve but she did not know how to do this.
11. Dupuytren's contractures were noted, flexing her ring and little fingers.

TREATMENT AIM

The treatment aim was now seen as a need to go back to the beginning by starting with trunk rehabilitation, exercises to be done on the sitting room floor (see mat work), and to introduce pressure splints and pressure techniques in an attempt to reverse the disabilities that had developed after the stroke over a period of 2 years. To reverse quite severe disabilities 2 years after the onset of a stroke is not an easy task; it takes time, dedication, continuing motivation and usually strong back-up.

A few initial home visits confirmed that the necessary back-up would be given by the patient's husband. Slowly, stage by stage, it was hoped that progress would be made in the recovery of lost function if pressure splints were used. The treatment concept presented in this book had not previously been tried. Husband and wife would work as a team; he would be taught to use the inflatable splints and to assist in the exercise routines. The visiting physiotherapist would go to their home once or twice a week to teach the advancing recovery routines and to show how to stabilize the starting position for each exercise progression.

If patients have no objection to the taking of photographs this can be a useful way of charting progress because it is not always easy to remember exactly how much progress has been made from month to month. It was hoped that as recovery went ahead the physiotherapist would gradually withdraw her support. In the beginning much of her teaching would concentrate on the use of inhibitory positioning and movement patterns, teaching the patient how to position and care for her own limbs and, once set up with the necessary inflation splints, how to take over the exercise routines by herself and reduce her husband's required supervision.

All went according to plan. Soon she was no longer nervous of being left in the house alone; she could be left on the floor to practise exercise routines while her husband did the household shopping. Later she almost became obsessed with the urgent need to exercise and she had to be taught that rest in inhibiting patterns was equally important. Because she recovered postural balance she lost her fear of going out of the house into the street supported by her husband – on her affected side! Later she went out alone, and she even boarded a bus alone. Her husband returned to the golf course; they could function together or separately; their quality of life was good. 'Thank you for giving us back our lives', was the telling comment he made to the physiotherapist.

The photographs (Figs 61–115) speak for themselves. They were taken over a period of 2 years and are presented here with full permission of the patient and her husband. They hope the pictures will be a help for other people.

Figures 61–66 were taken over a period of 24 months (1992–1994) at intervals of 4 months and are an excellent series to be used for assessment purposes. The patient is standing and has been asked to lift both hands above her head with her palms facing each other.

Figure 61 shows a severely disabled left arm and also shows that she apparently has some degree of trunk spasticity with trunk shortening on her disabled side. The patient appears not to be fully weightbearing on her disabled side, and manual examination very soon demonstrated the fairly typical problems of an immobile scapula with retracted and inwardly rotated shoulder joint and flexor spasticity of elbow, wrist and fingers. Her face seems to register disgust as she looks at the hand which she cannot control. A thorough assessment was undertaken and the results noted as above.

An attempt would be made to shift abnormal tonal patterns back to normal and restore normal movement. Pressure techniques would be used to maintain inhibitory patterns and to divert tonal flow into the recovery pattern, at the same time increasing sensory input. Motor developmental patterns would be used.

By the time Figure 63 was taken, 10 months after treatment with pressure splints was started, it was safe to begin to believe that rehabilitation would have a successful outcome.

As soon as treatment was started the immediate priorities were established as follows:

1. To teach the patient's husband to apply the long arm inflatable pressure splint.
2. To start manual mobilization of the trunk and shoulder.
3. To stabilize the patient lying on her back with both knees bent up, i.e. the crook lying position, or the starting position for bridging. At first the affected knee flopped outward into outward rotation of the hip. Active assisted work into inward rotation of the hip was given and stabilizing techniques were used. This was carried out with the long arm splint controlling the tonal pattern in the arm.

The following photographs illustrate just some of the exercise routines that were used.

Figs 61–66 are a photographic record of improvement in the hemiplegic arm over a period of 2 years. These are useful assessment records showing progress in the recovery process.

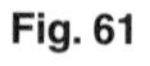

Fig. 61

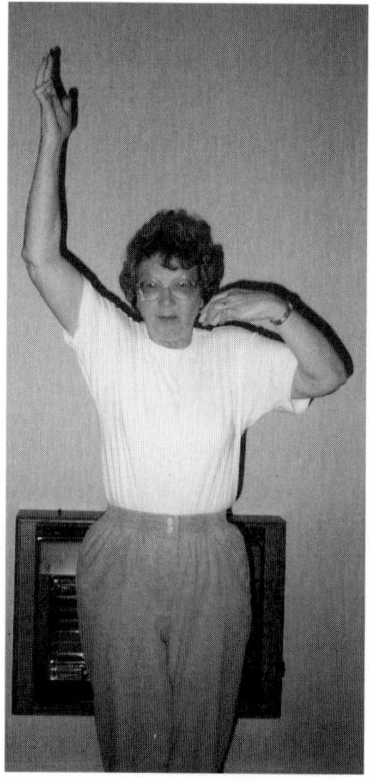

Fig. 62

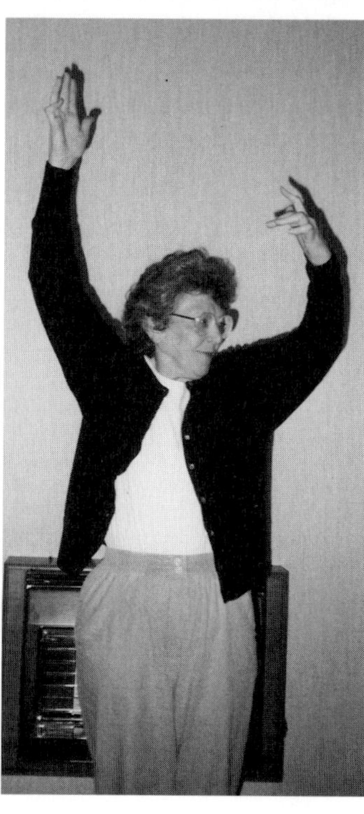

Fig. 63

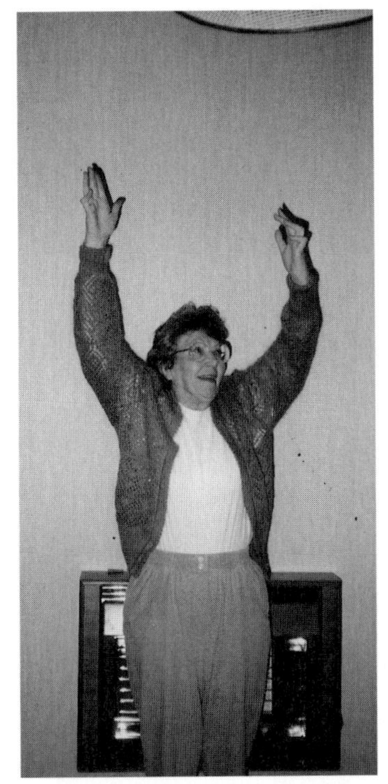

Fig. 64

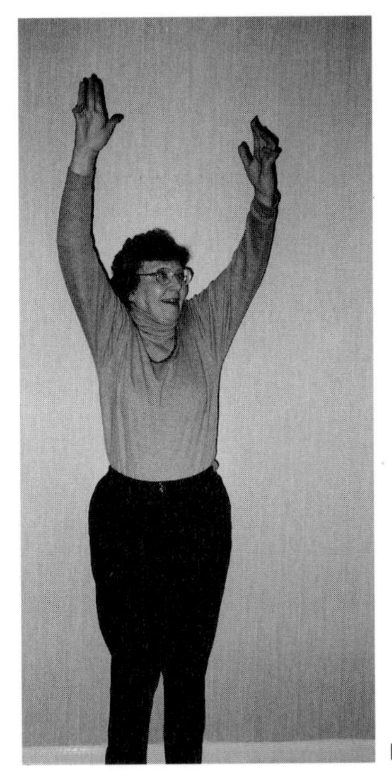

Fig. 65

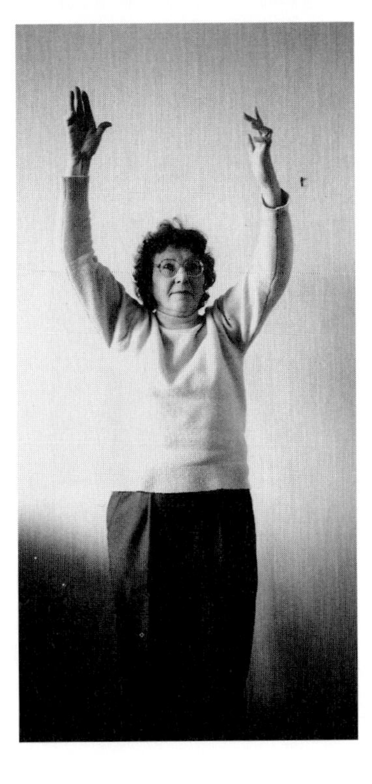

Fig. 66

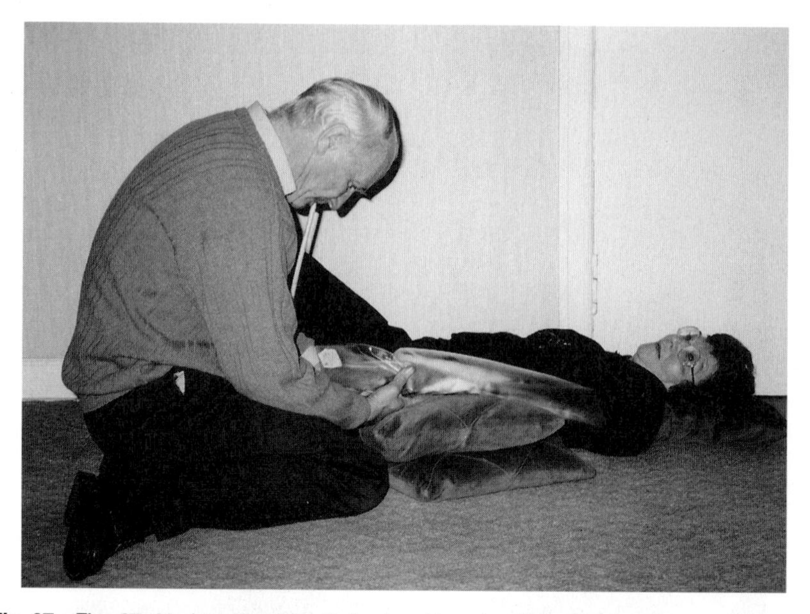

Fig. 67 Figs 67–68 show the patient's husband learning to apply the splint.

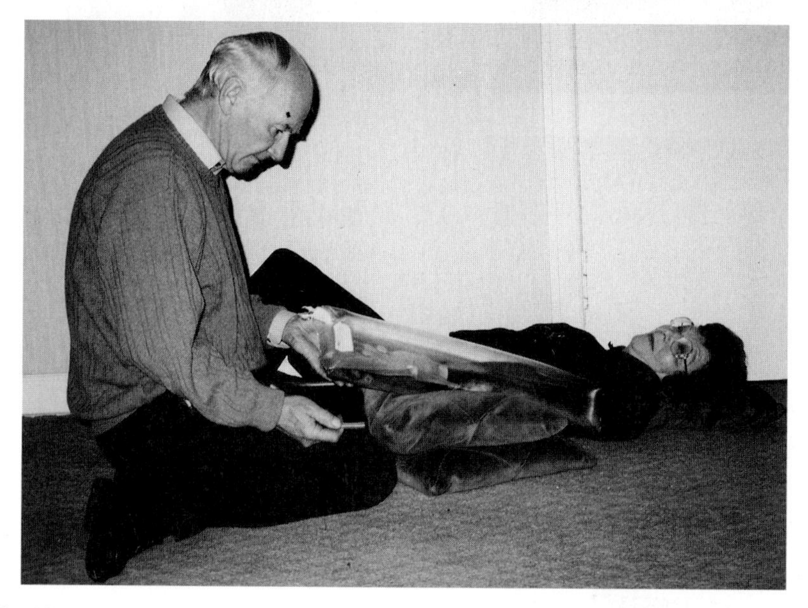

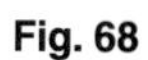

Fig. 68

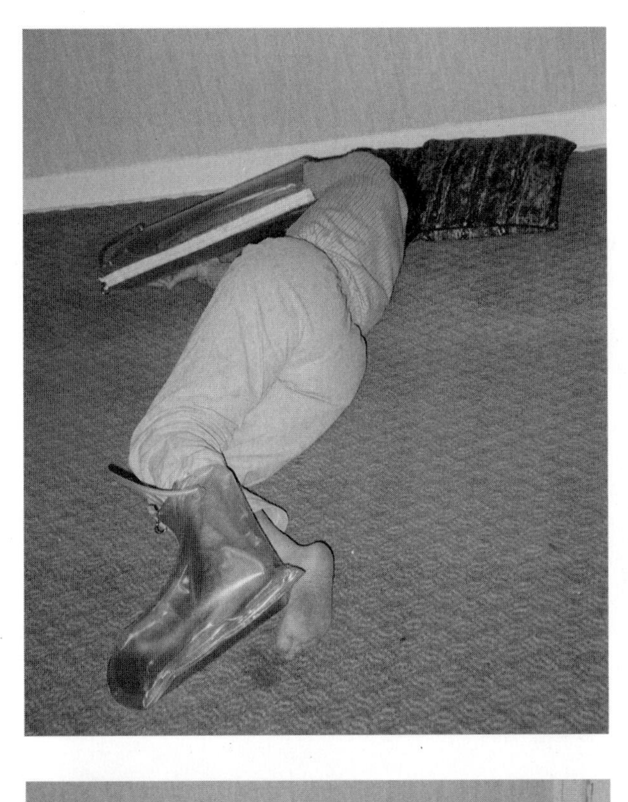

Fig. 69
Figs 69–70 show rolling from side to side. Lead the movement with eyes and head turning in the direction of the roll, followed by trunk rotation with the sound arm assisting the splinted arm.

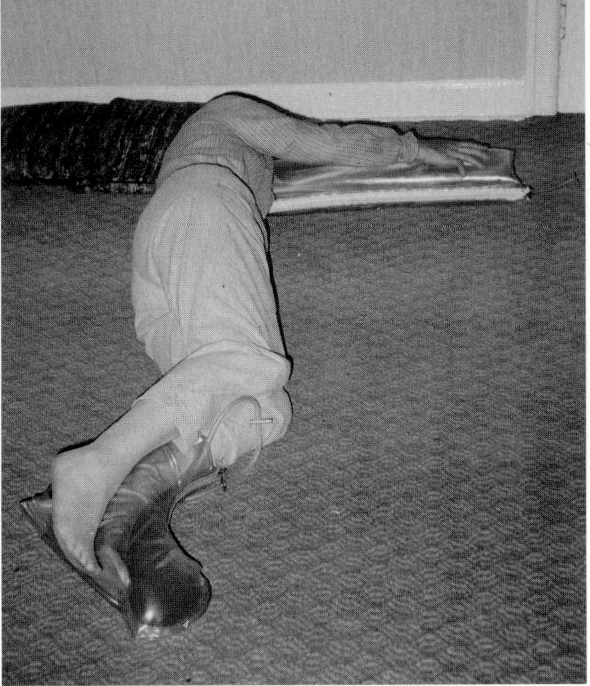

Fig. 70

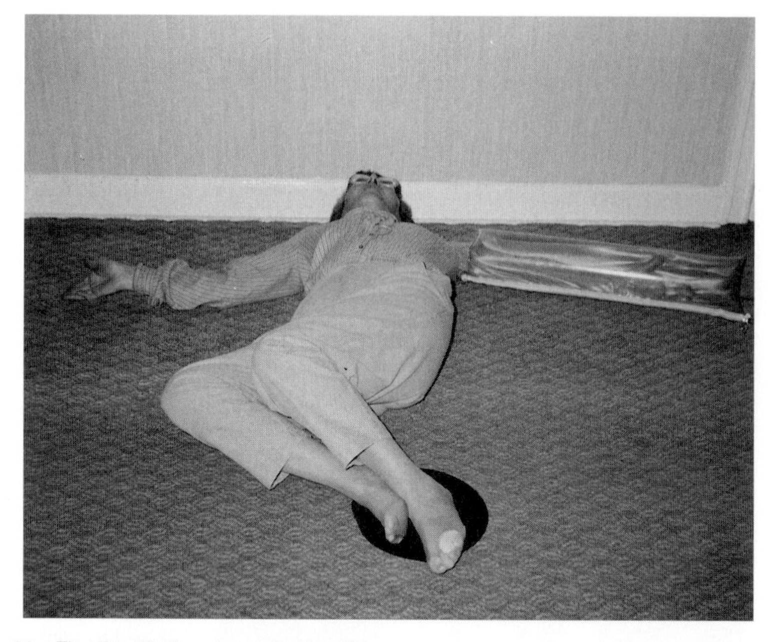

Fig. 71 Figs 71–72 show lower trunk rolling.

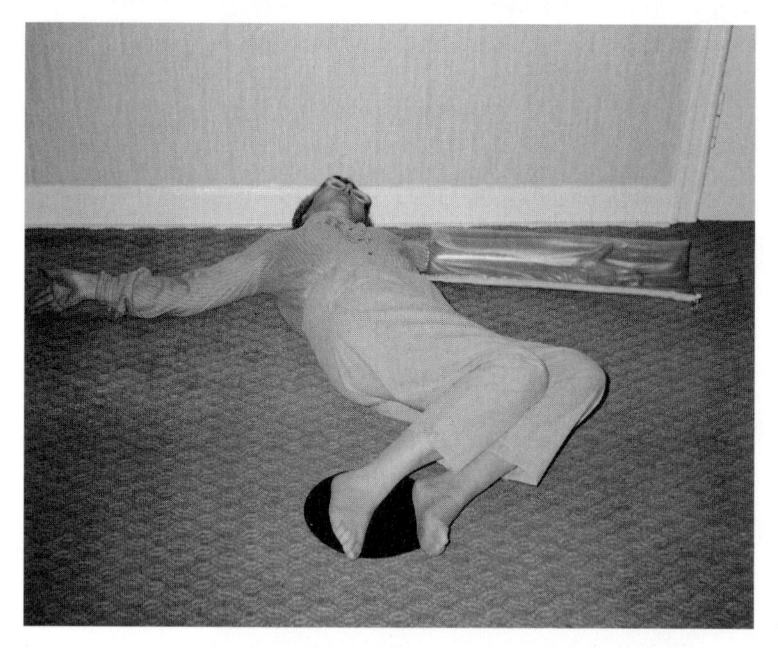

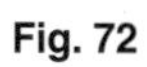

Fig. 72

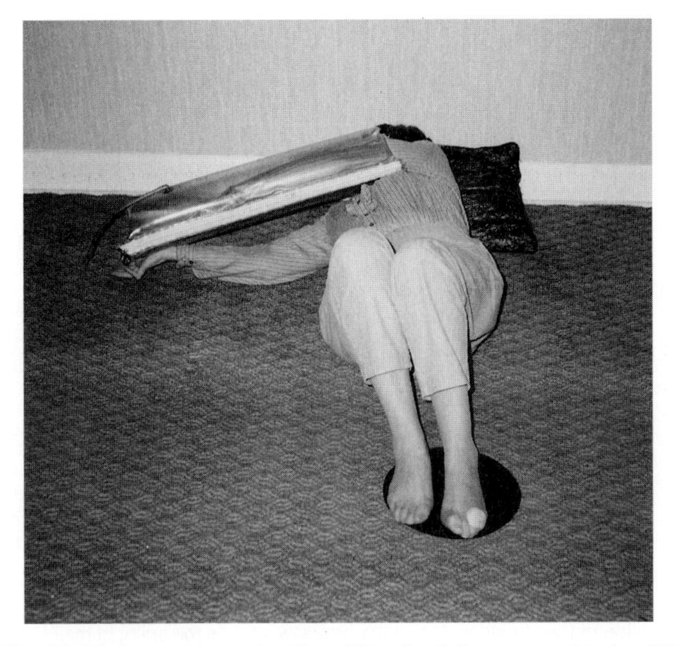

Fig. 73 Figs 73–74 show upper trunk rolling. All trunk rotations are assisted until the patient can maintain the inhibiting patterns and go it alone.

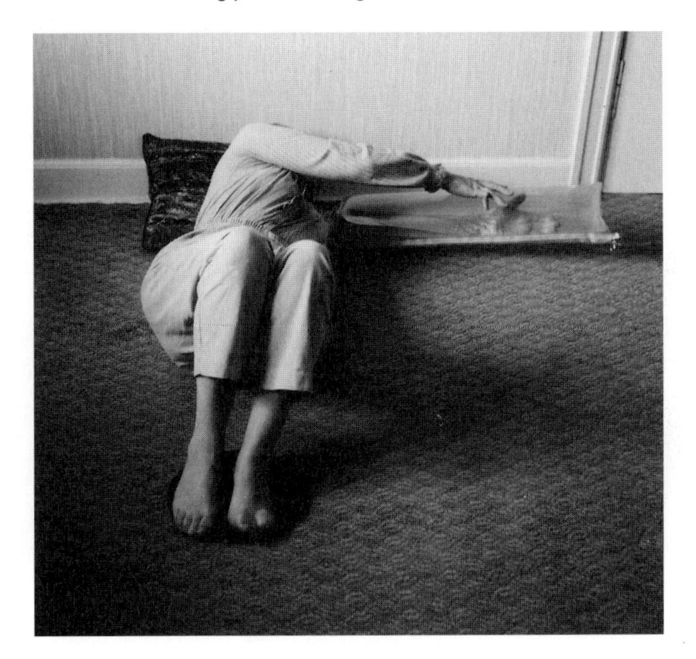

Fig. 74

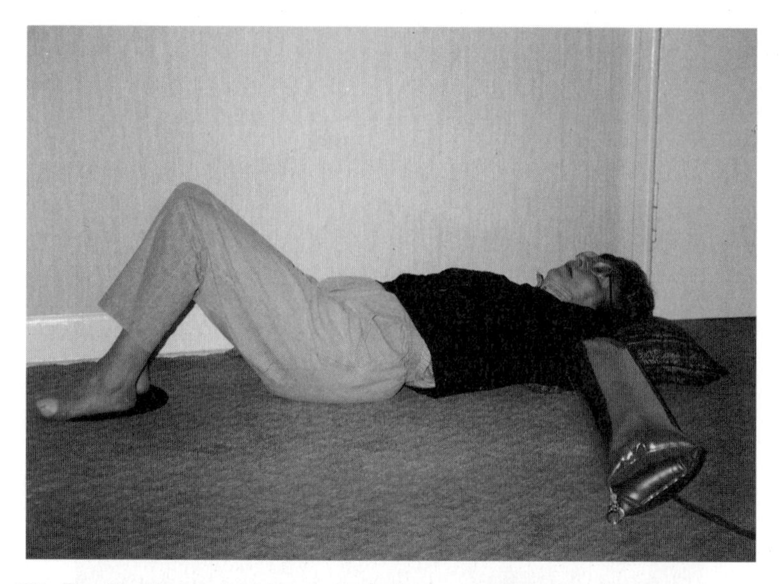

Fig. 75 Figs 75–76 show bridging. As the buttocks are lifted off the floor there is a strong flow of tone into the arm. The pressure splint diverts this into the full inhibiting pattern of outward rotation of the shoulder. At first the operator assists the splint in maintaining the corrective pattern; later, as recovery advances, help is no longer necessary, and the splinted arm can be seen to roll into stronger outward rotation as the buttocks are lifted.

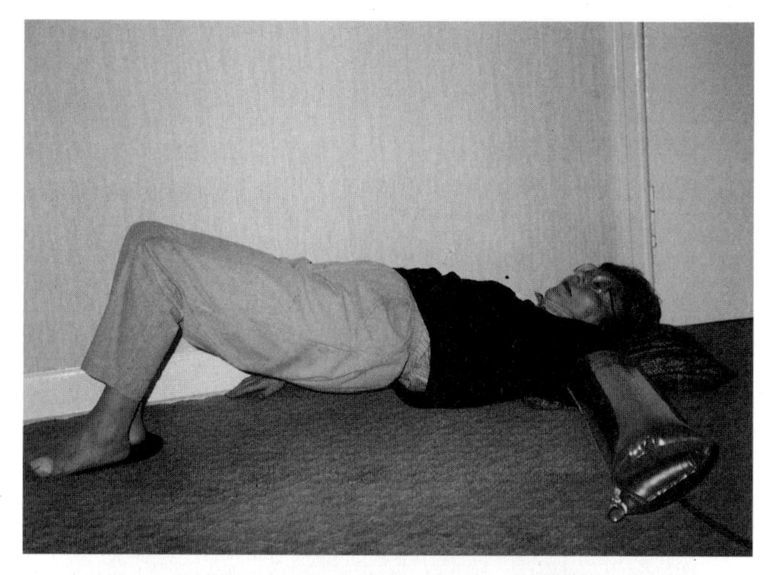

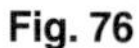

Fig. 76

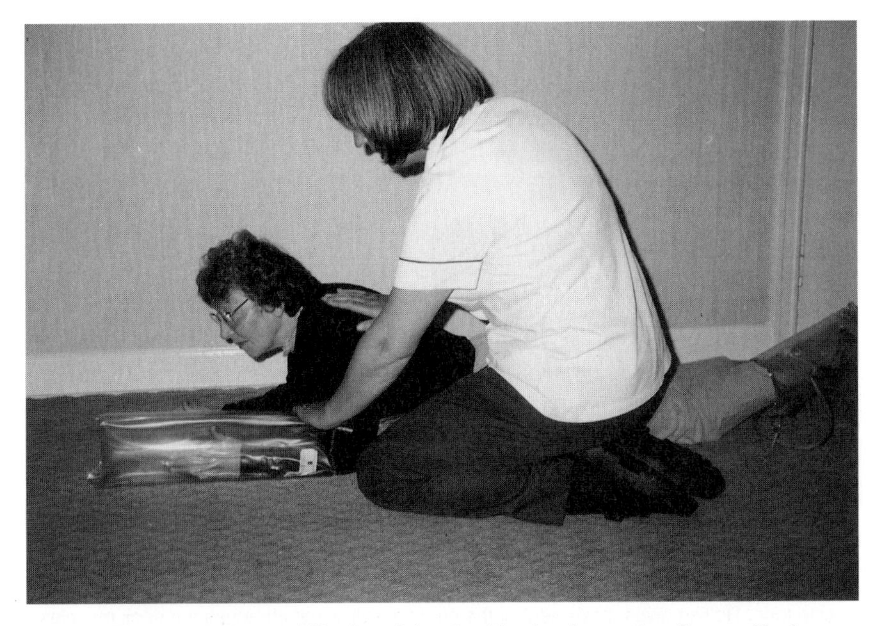

Fig. 77 Figs 77–78 show stabilization of the shoulder, leaning on the elbows with ulna border leaning on parallel forearms. The physiotherapist demonstrates to the family carer how to increase the input by increasing the downward pressure through the shoulder. She also uses the tonic neck extension response by asking the patient to lift her head backwards against pressure. A mirror placed at eye level can increase this response as the patient lifts her head to look at her mirror image.

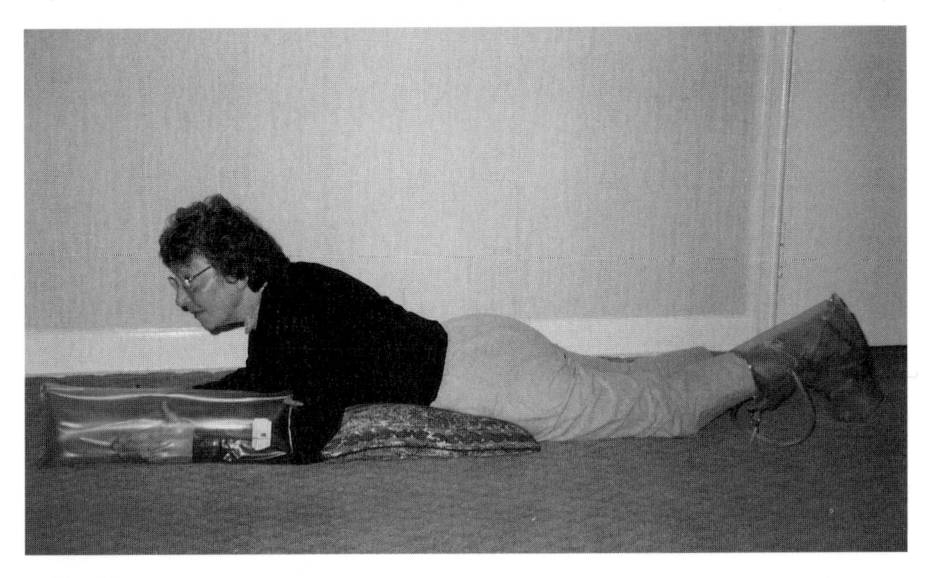

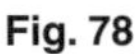

Fig. 78

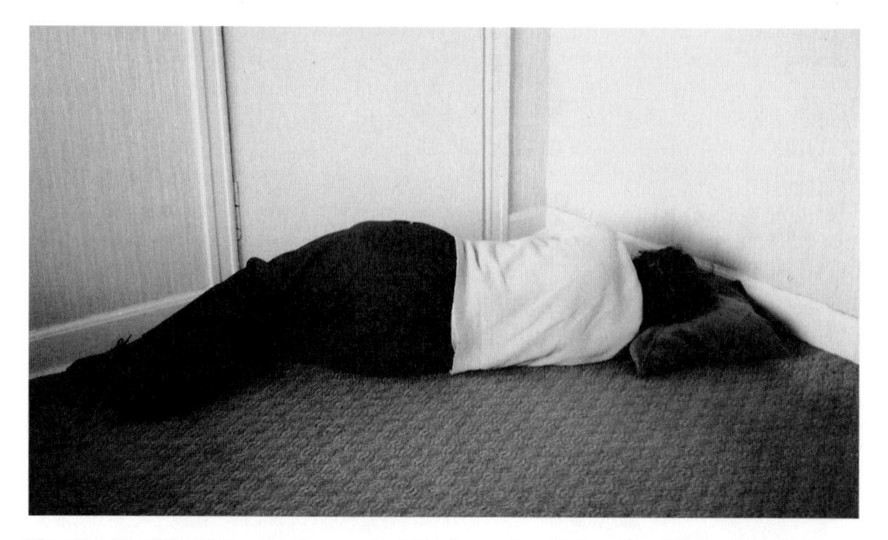

Fig. 79 Figs 79–82 represent a very important exercise progression. The patient clasps her hands, palms touching, and rolls over and over across the floor, keeping elbows straight, at or above shoulder level. The position of the head has a fundamental bearing on muscle tone. Rolling gives movement of the cervical spine and stretches the neck muscles. This triggers off the reflex mechanism to bring the body into alignment of head, neck and trunk. This leads to controlled rolling, controlled rolling to sitting, and finally to the ability to rotate about the body axis and therefore to controlled movement, rotation being a necessary component of normal movement.

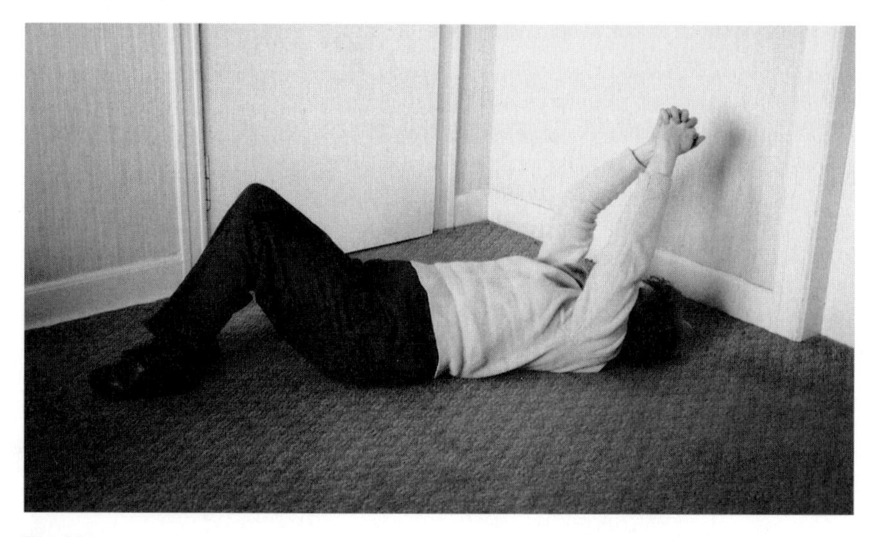

Fig. 80

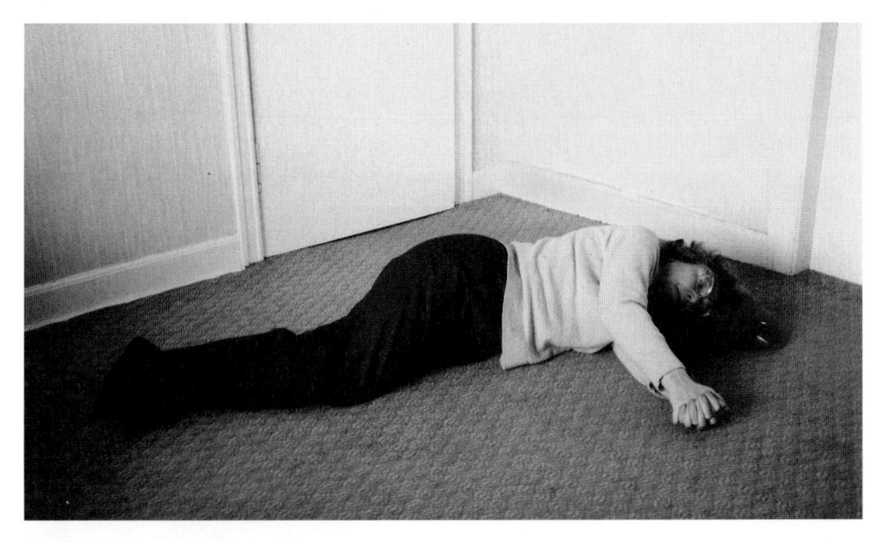

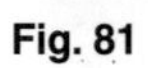

Fig. 81

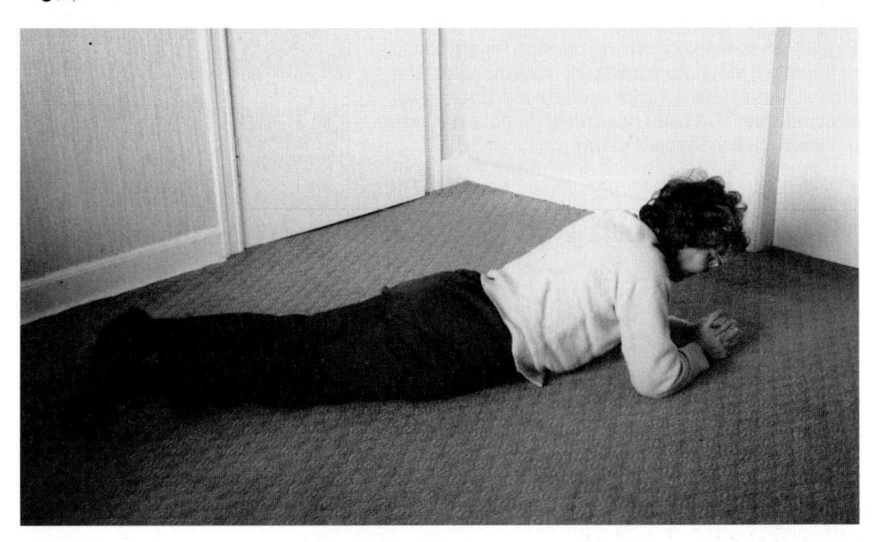

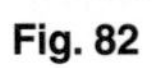

Fig. 82

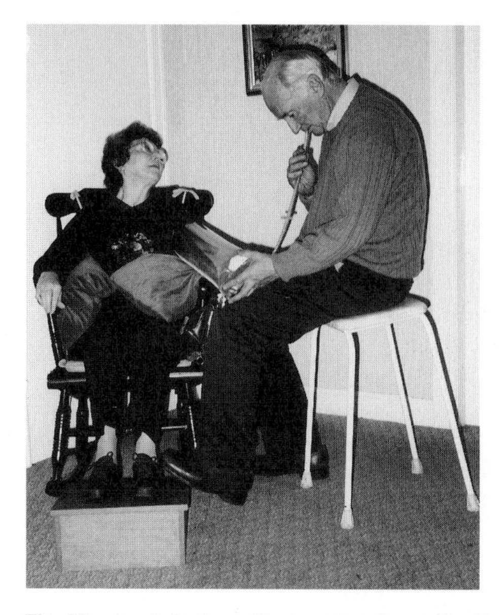

Fig. 83 A satisfactory sitting position for application of the arm splint before using the rocking chair. The patient's head is tilted back and rotated towards her affected side. The head position influences corrective tonal distribution in the forearm.

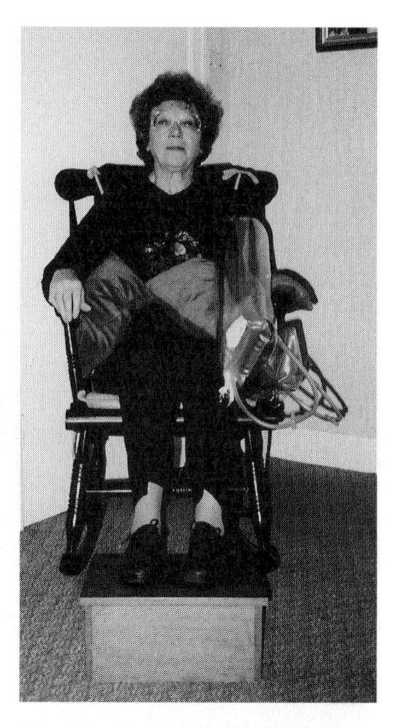

Fig. 84 An excellent inhibitory sitting position. Music can motivate the rocking movement.

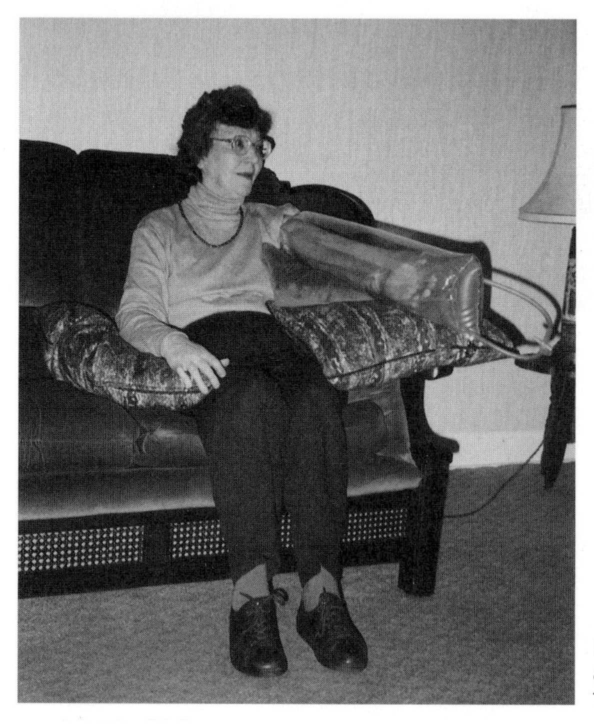

Fig. 85 The therapeutic approach to watching television.

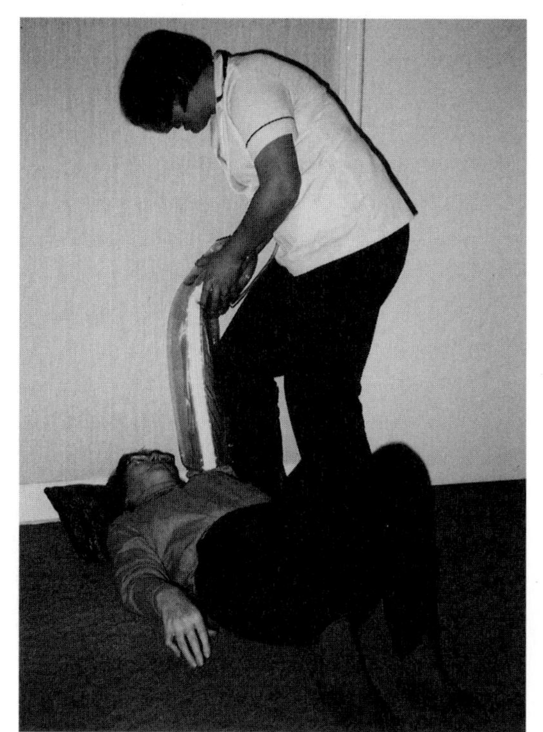

Fig. 86 Figs 86–87: 'Reach for the ceiling!'. Shoulder protraction against resistance on an extended wrist with outward rotation of the shoulder. Graduate the resistance carefully.

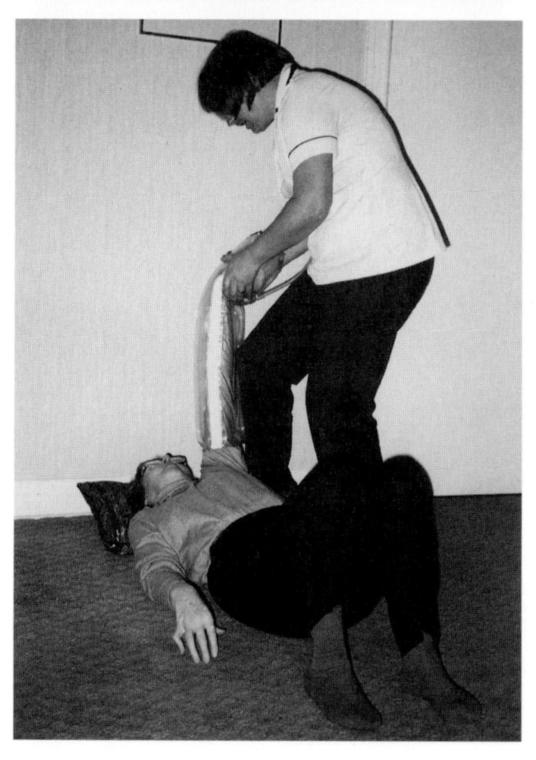

Fig. 87

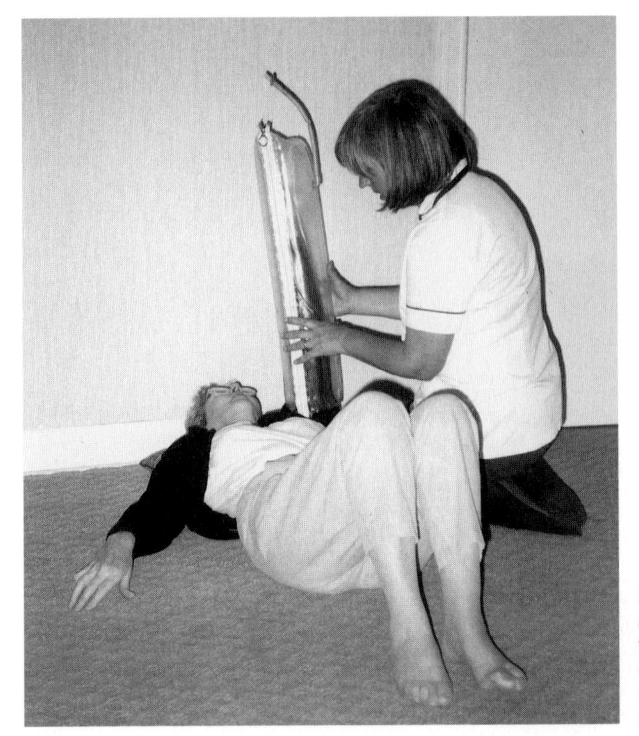

Fig. 88 Figs 88–89: a placing response in the shoulder has been achieved with the pressure splint giving arm stability.

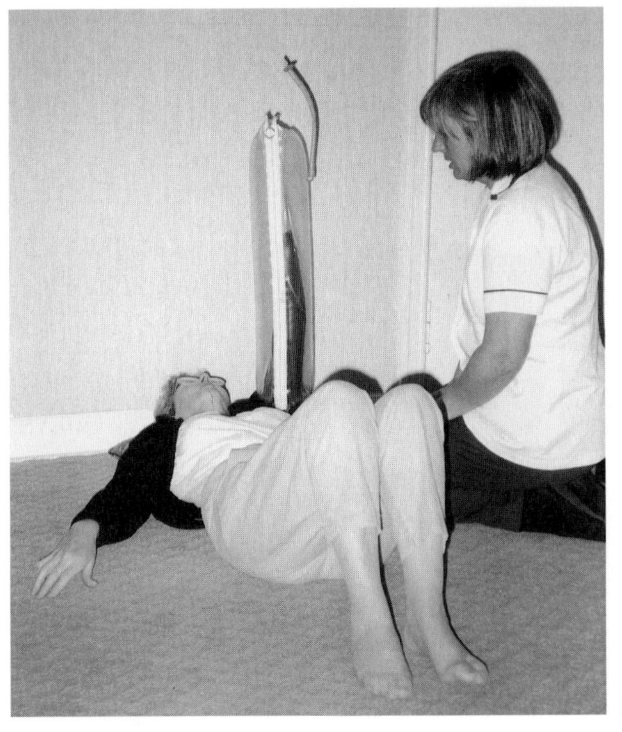

Fig. 89

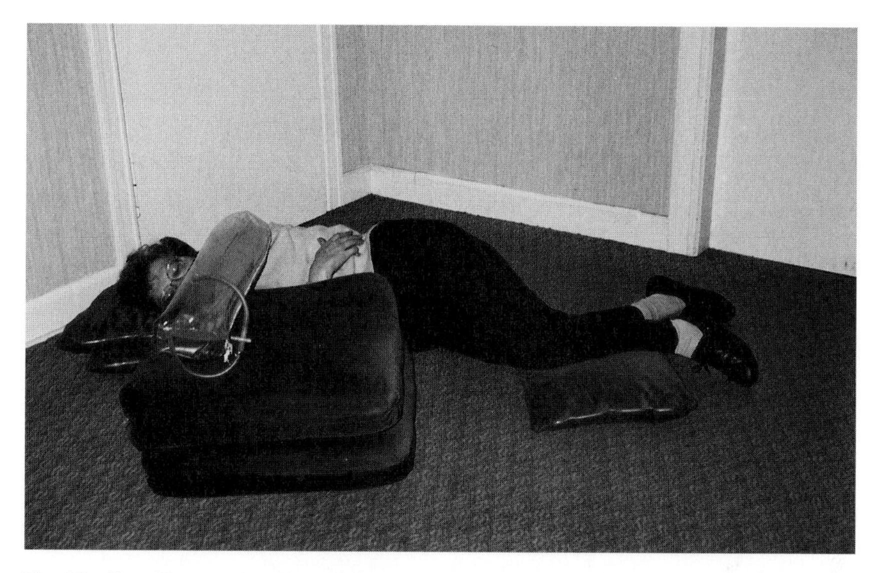

Fig. 90 Figs 90–91: using the splinted arm as a saw, the patient attempts to 'saw the cushion in half!'. An example of a self-care exercise. The rehabilitation programme concentrates on encouraging the use of self-care exercise.

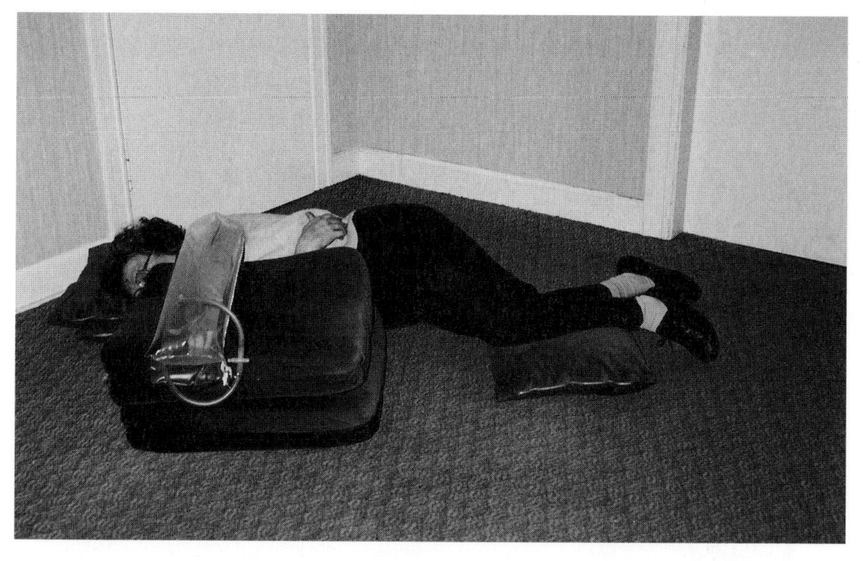

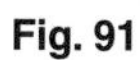

Fig. 91

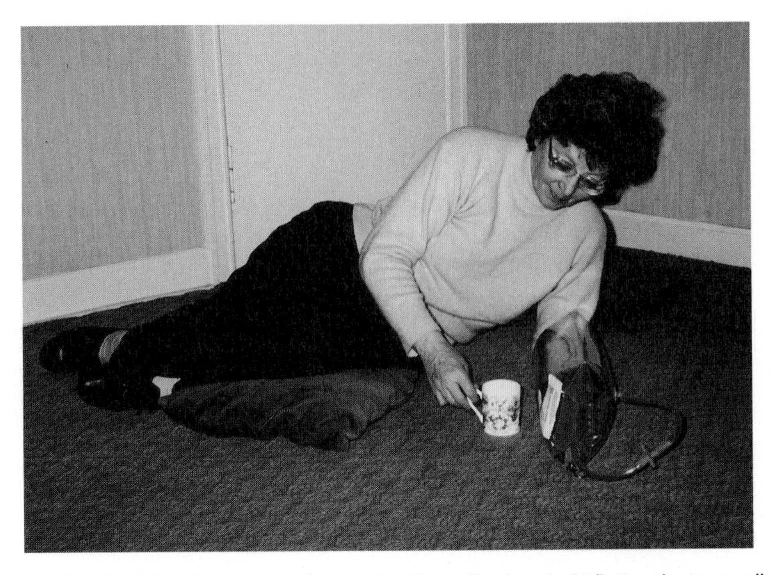

Fig. 92 Figs 92–93: self-care exercise used in the coffee break. At first patients usually need assistance to get the forearm into the correct position, so that weight is distributed from forearm to shoulder, with the shoulder directly above the elbow and in an acceptable position of outward rotation.

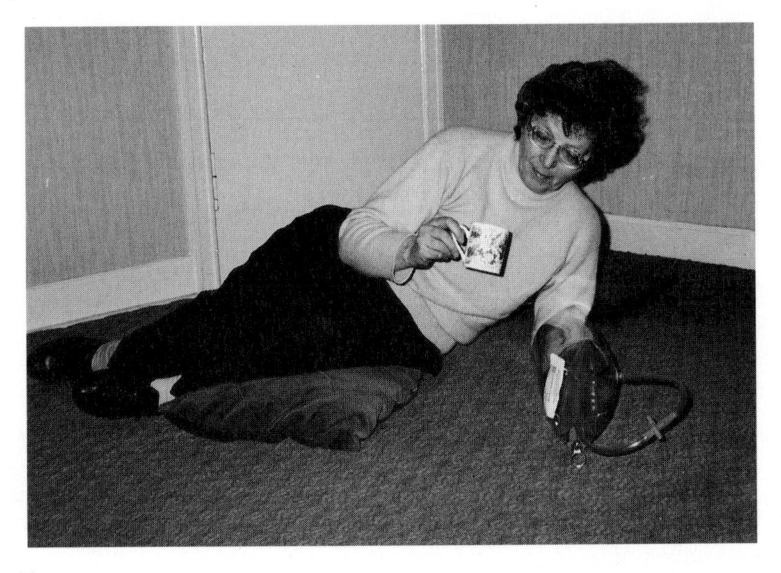

Fig. 93

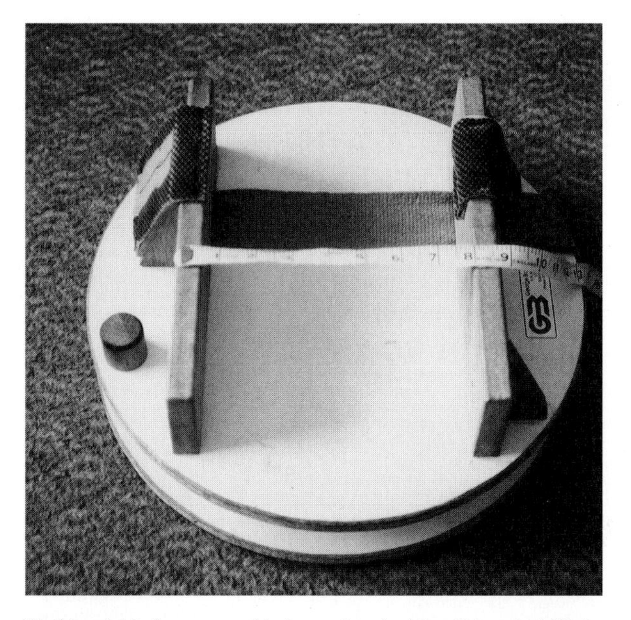

Fig. 94 The Wolf turntable has proved to be an invaluable aid to rehabilitation of the hemiplegic arm. The tape-measure shows the distance between the uprights. Use the peg when a static base is needed, and remove it when movement into outward rotation is required. (For further details about the turntable, see the Appendix.)

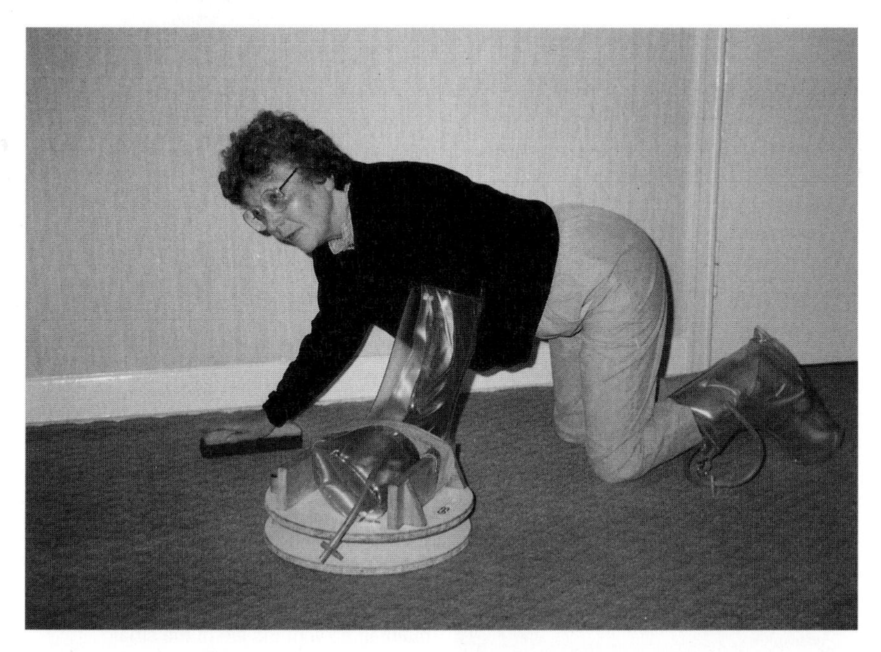

Fig. 95 The arm still lacks stability. Get extensor tone into the elbow by helping to support the arm in the full inhibiting position with reinforced elbow extension. The best way to increase tone in any limb is to put weight through it, but make sure the full inhibiting pattern is used.

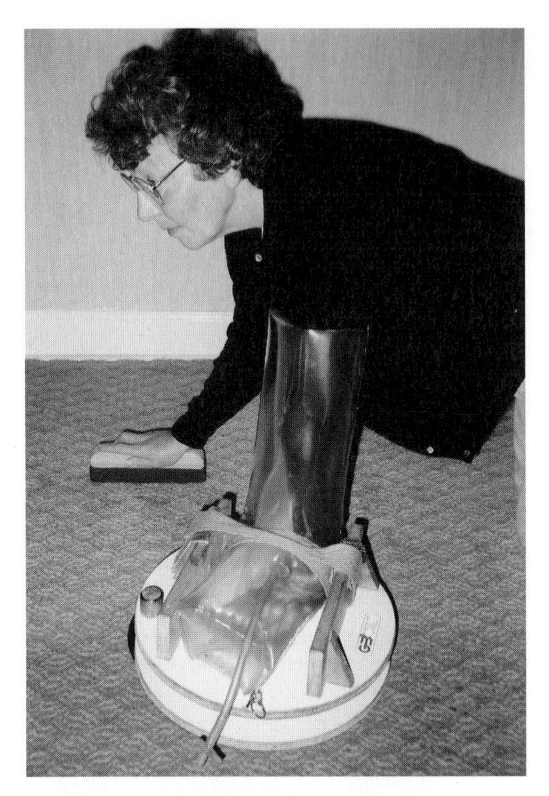

Fig. 96 Arm stability is now established, and the patient is ready to start crawling. The static base controlling the inhibited hand position is now converted into the useful turntable by removing the large wooden peg, and the patient is taught to crawl round the inhibited arm.

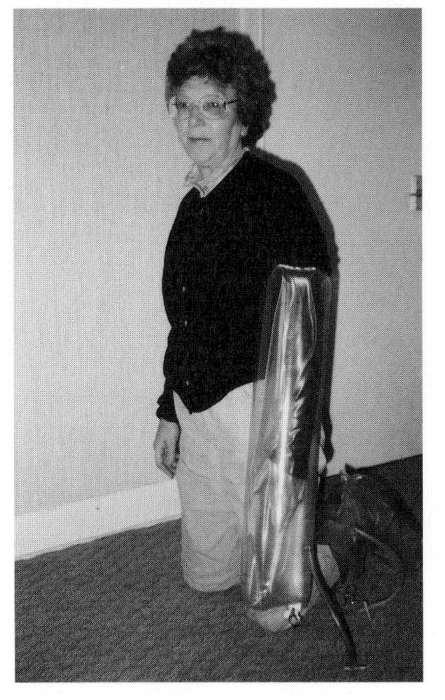

Fig. 97 In the advancing rehabilitation programme, standing balance on the knees is achieved while the inhibiting pattern is maintained with the aid of the small pressure boot. This position should be thoroughly stabilized. In the case of osteoarthritic knees, see Fig. 36, and use a kneeling cushion plus long arm splint.

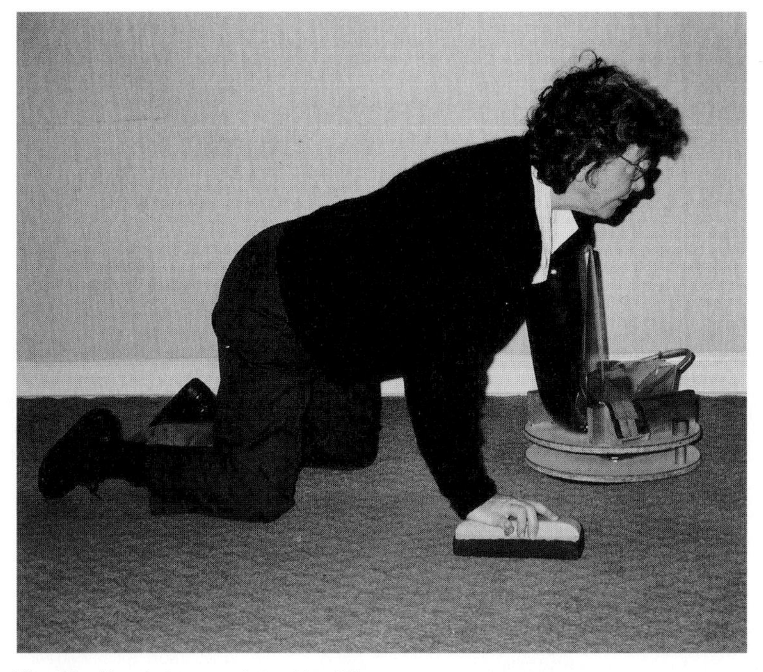

Fig. 98 Ready to move into side sitting.

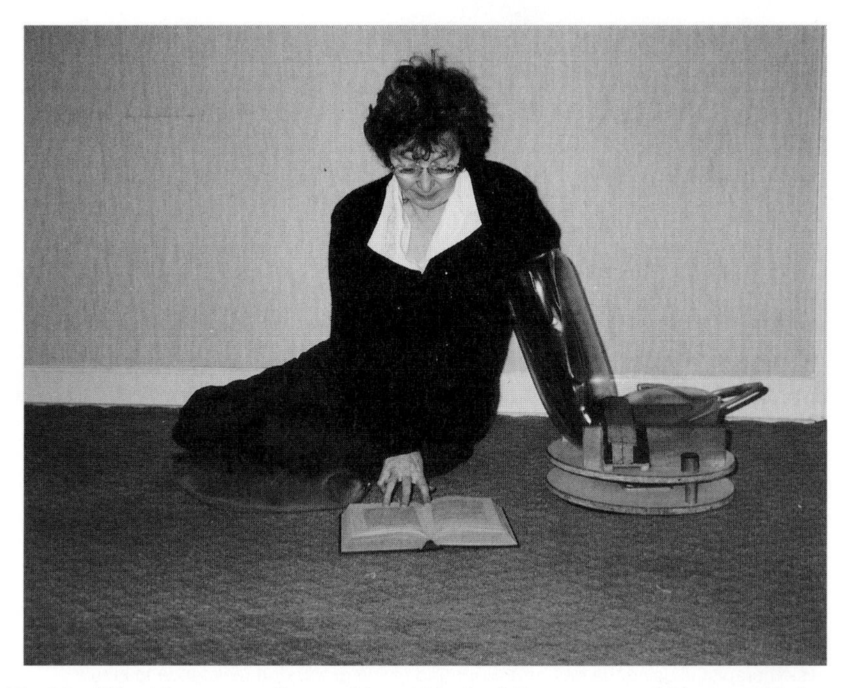

Fig. 99 Side sitting; an excellent position which should be encouraged. The turntable is again fixed with the wooden peg. Note the pillow helping to maintain inward rotation of the thigh.

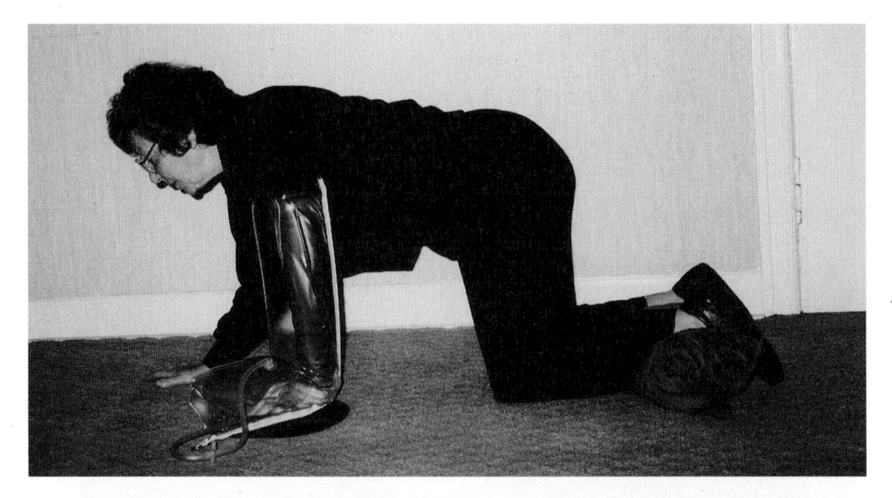

Fig. 100 Figs 100–101: crawling positions are used and the patient is encouraged to do self-care exercises, e.g. Fig. 100: both hands on the floor, rocking backwards and forwards over the hands.

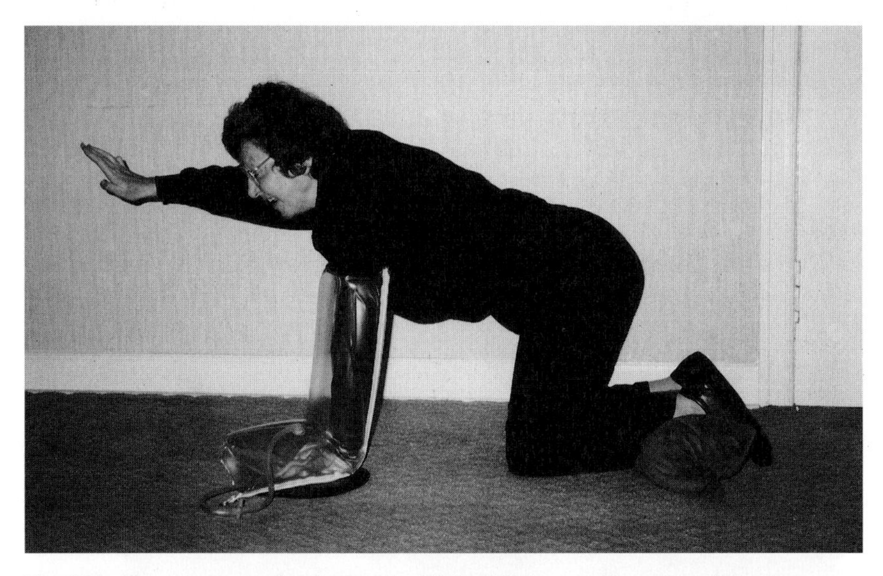

Fig. 101 The patient must be thoroughly stabilized in the crawling pattern (see also Fig. 100) and advancing balance training is introduced by progressive exercise patterns, e.g. as shown here. Stretching alternate legs backwards into extension may also be used.

Figs 102–104 show a method for training strong elbow extension to build up triceps. The physiotherapist is using the half-arm splint and giving graduated resistance to elbow extension. Passive and active supination of the forearm was also encouraged and difficult to establish. The supinator muscle seemed non-existent and the memory of movement into supination was missing. *This movement should be trained from the very early days.*

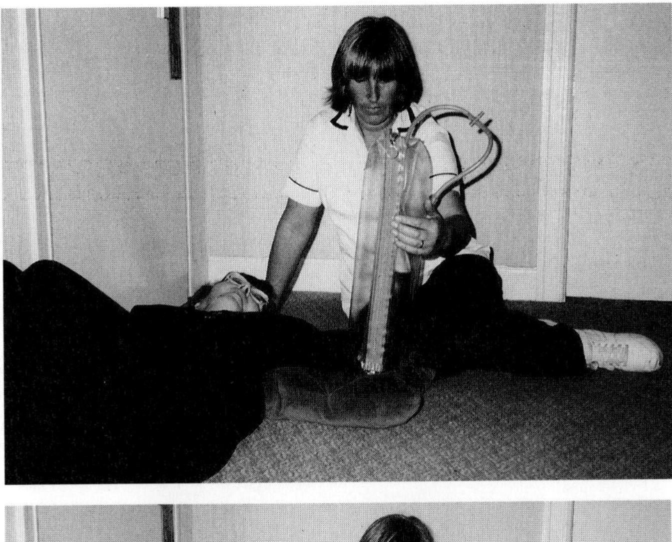

Fig. 102

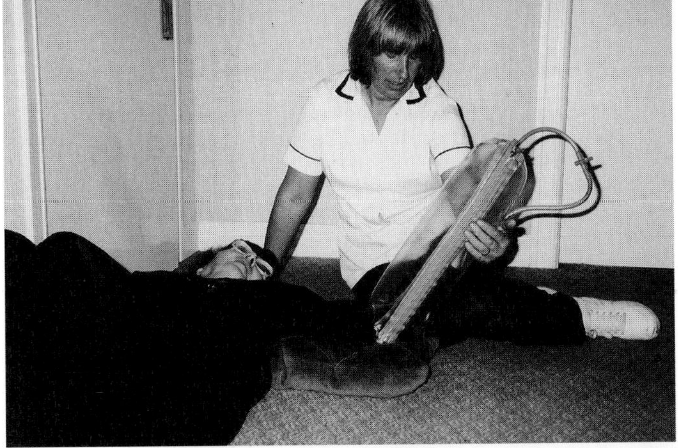

Fig. 103

Fig. 104

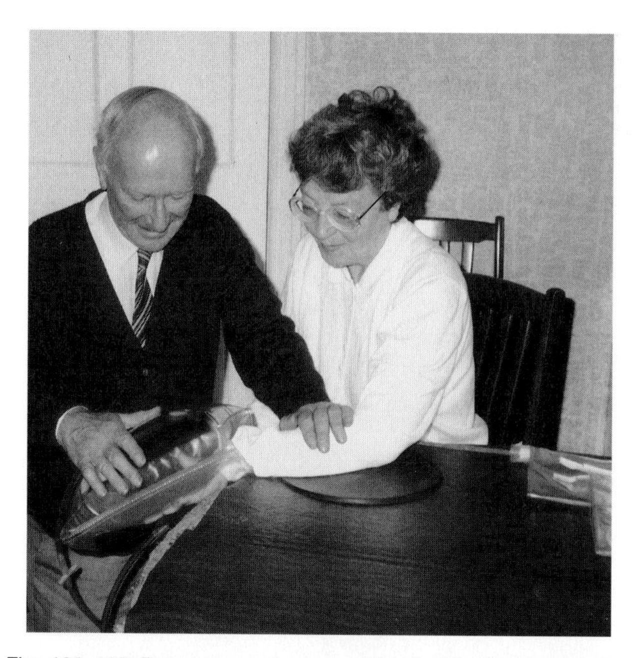

Fig. 105 Figs 105–106: Recovery continues, and the double chamber hand splint is brought into use. Remember to inflate the section over the back of the hand first, to bring in extensor response. Then add a little air to the front section. Here graduated resistance is given to the back of the hand to build up wrist extension.

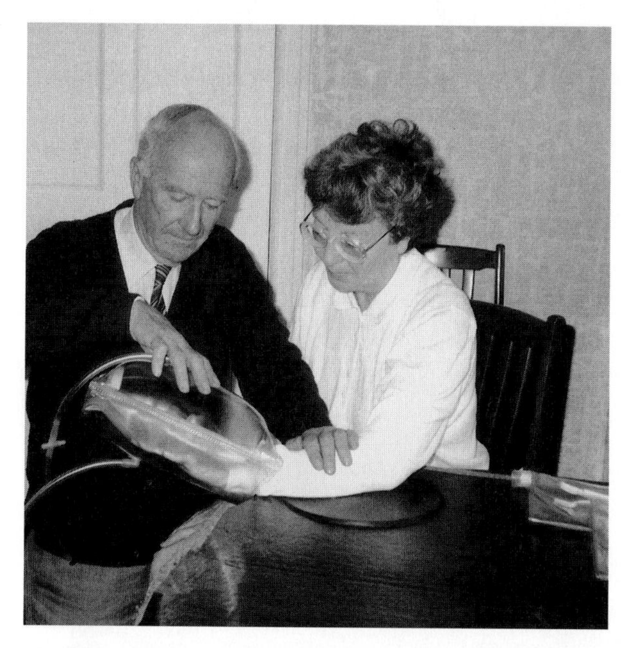

Fig. 106

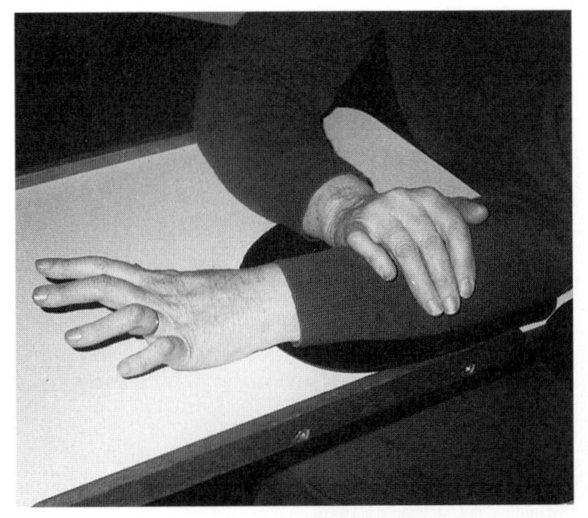

Fig. 107 Taking the Dupuytren's contracture into account (which, comparing this with earlier photos, has improved with the use of the splints), it is agreed that recovery of hand function is going well.

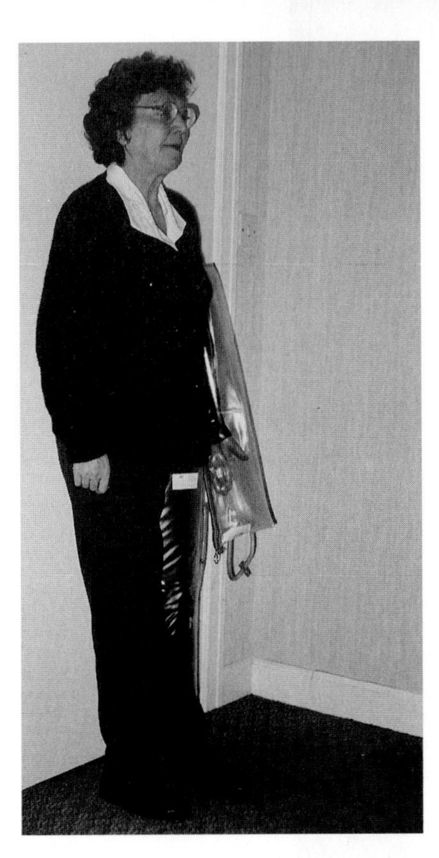

Fig. 108

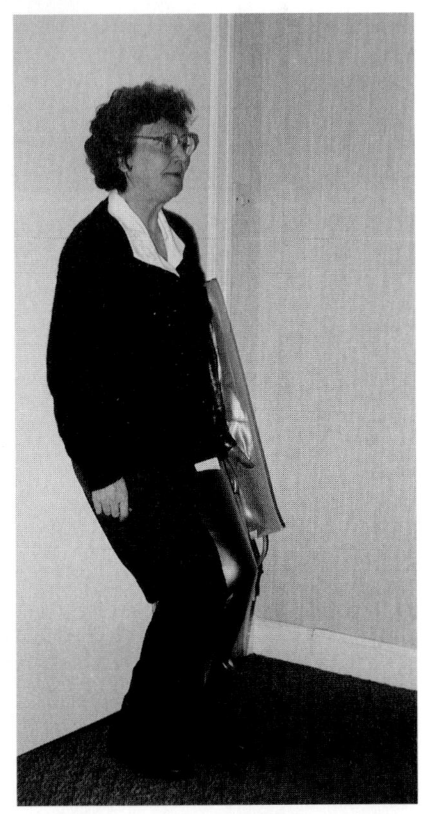

Fig. 109

Figs 108–109: 'squat sits' are used to boost leg recovery. With the leg gaiter correctly applied to bring in knee flexion, the patient stands with heels firmly on the floor, and feet pointing straight forward. She leans backwards to support her back against the door, and, bending and stretching her knees, she slides up and down the door.

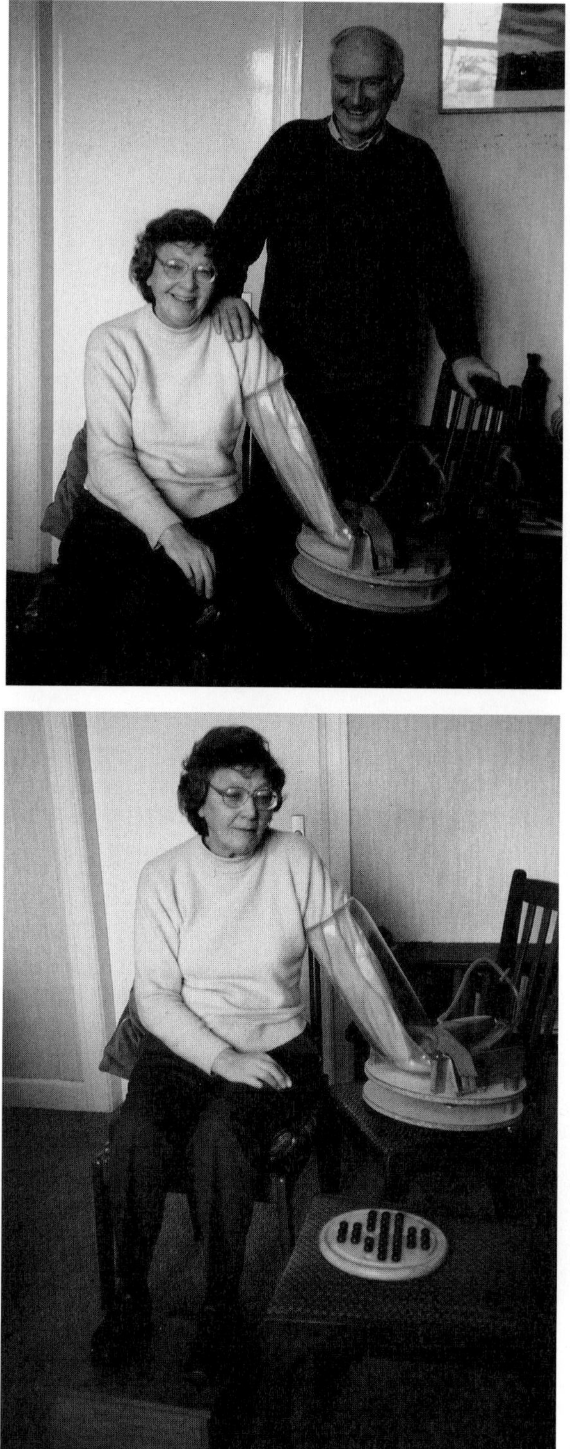

Fig. 110 Figs 110–111: life begins to look good again!

Fig. 111

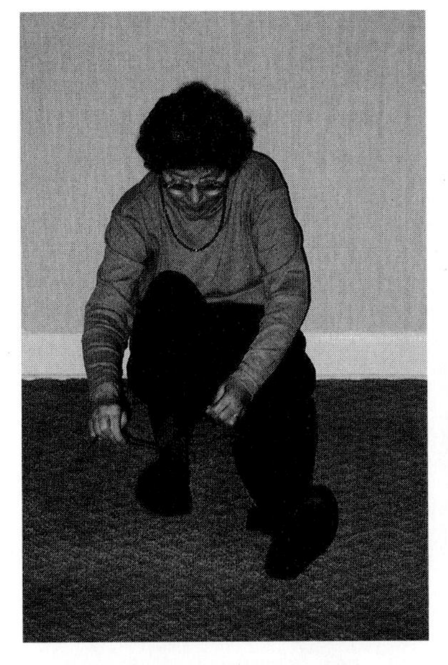

Fig. 112 Figs 112–113: recovery of fine finger control; the patient tying her shoelaces.

Fig. 113

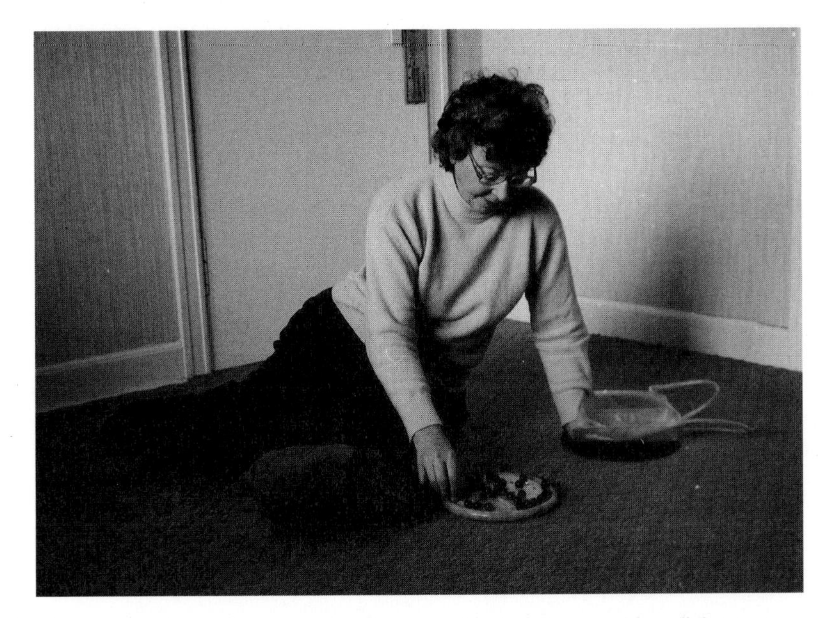

Fig. 114 The patient continues to exercise daily. She feels the need for a little more strength in the recovered arm.

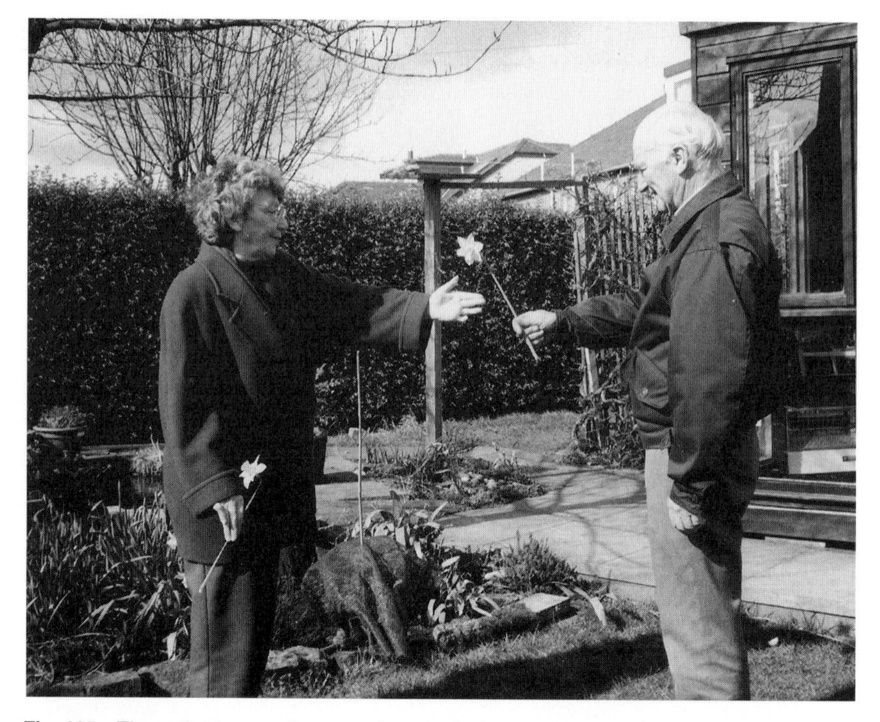

Fig. 115 The patient can walk on rough grass in the garden. Her husband asks her to reach for the flower he is presenting. She reaches and her arm and hand move into the completed recovery pattern, showing that normal muscle tone has been restored. Strong antigravity tone can no longer interfere to prevent normal movement. Cortical control has been re-established.

CASE HISTORY 2

The rehabilitation concept presented in this book is beginning to be disseminated more widely, and in recent years has been used with patients who have sustained neurological damage other than stroke. Figures 116–122, taken in the later stages of recovery, show one such patient. In Figures 116–121 he is shown using the 'Fitter' exerciser.

This patient sustained severe brain damage and multiple injuries in a car crash, and 17 months later he was still facing considerable physical problems, presenting with left hemiplegia and movement patterns which were dictated by spasticity. This included his trunk and both left limbs. He was now 31 years of age. In spite of help offered by conventional physiotherapy he was showing little or no progress. He was unable to contemplate anything like normal living.

At this stage it was vital to regain postural balance, if there was to be any chance of regaining normal movement. It was decided that the patient should be introduced to treatment with pressure splints and pressure techniques. His rehabilitation programme was transferred to a different venue, where the treatment concept presented in this book was offered.

Since then he has made slow but very steady progress, until now he is leading a full and independent life. He had a long and hard battle to reduce trunk spasticity, and this was followed by a return to normal balance reactions and steady improvement in the movement performance of his limbs. For example, he began to develop a heel strike in his walking gait. The further and final improvement in limb stability has now begun.

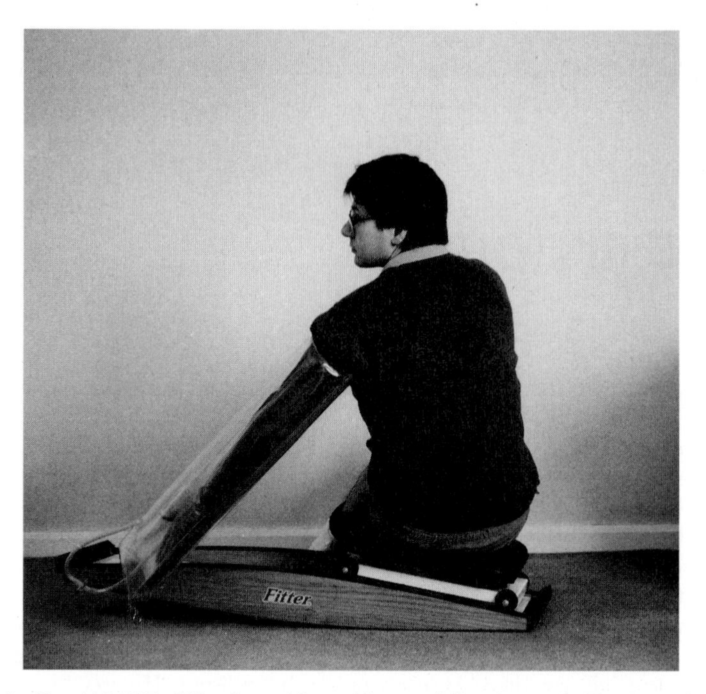

Fig. 116 Figs 116–117: sliding from side to side to mobilize the trunk. Elastic cords stretching from end to end, underneath, control the amount of resistance given to the movement. By this stage the patient has achieved enough independence to carry out his own exercise routines.

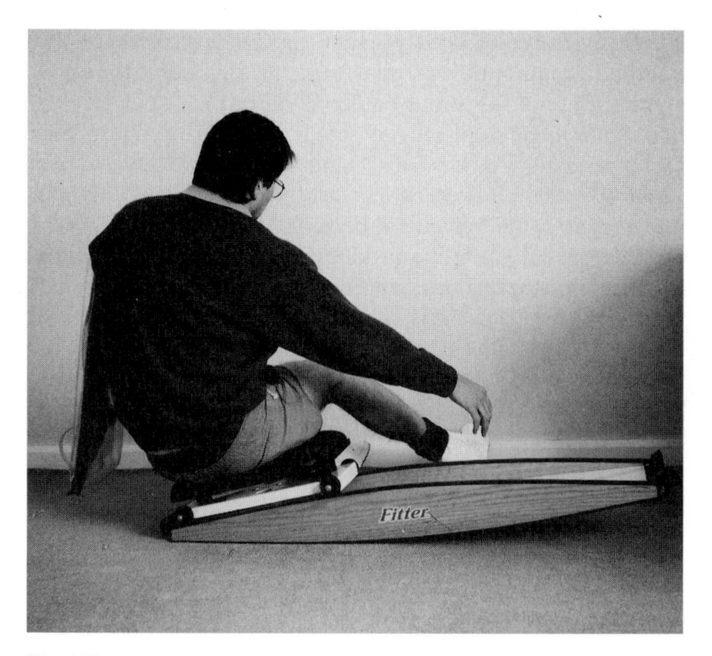

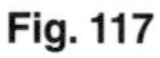

Fig. 117

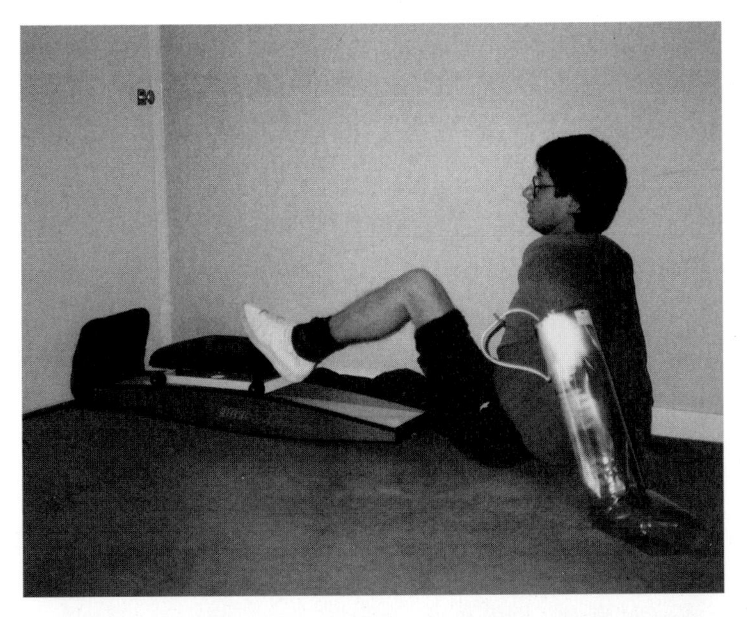

Fig. 118 Figs 118–119: working the quadriceps. The elastic cord resists the knee extension, and brings the seat, which is on wheels, back up the slope with knee extension. At the same time, with the inhibited arm position maintained by a pressure splint, arm treatment is given.

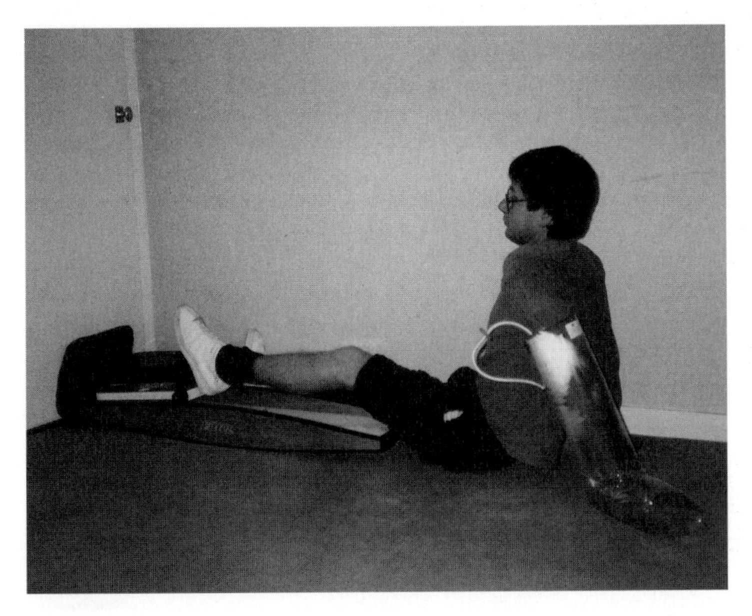

Fig. 119

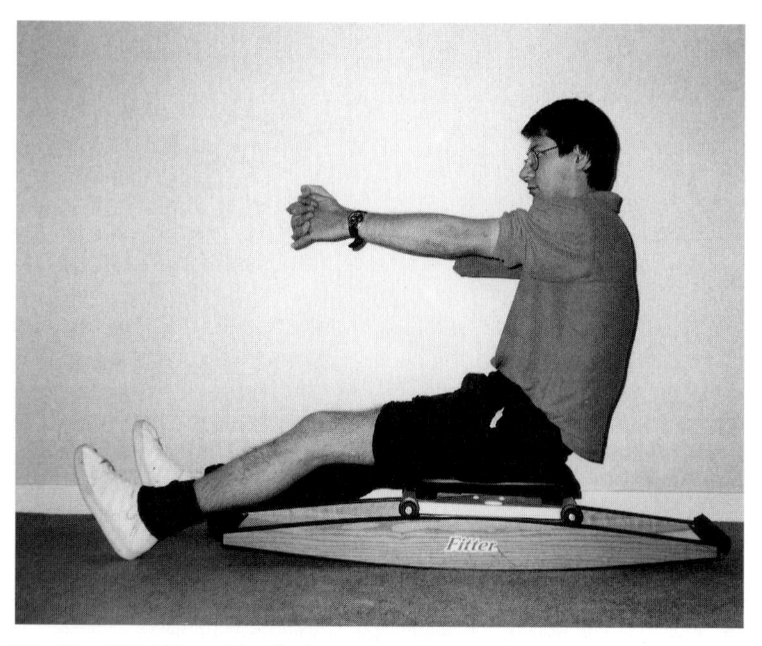

Fig. 120 Figs 120–121: working the hamstrings. Here, with knee flexion, the patient drags the seat down the slope against resistance from the elastic cord.

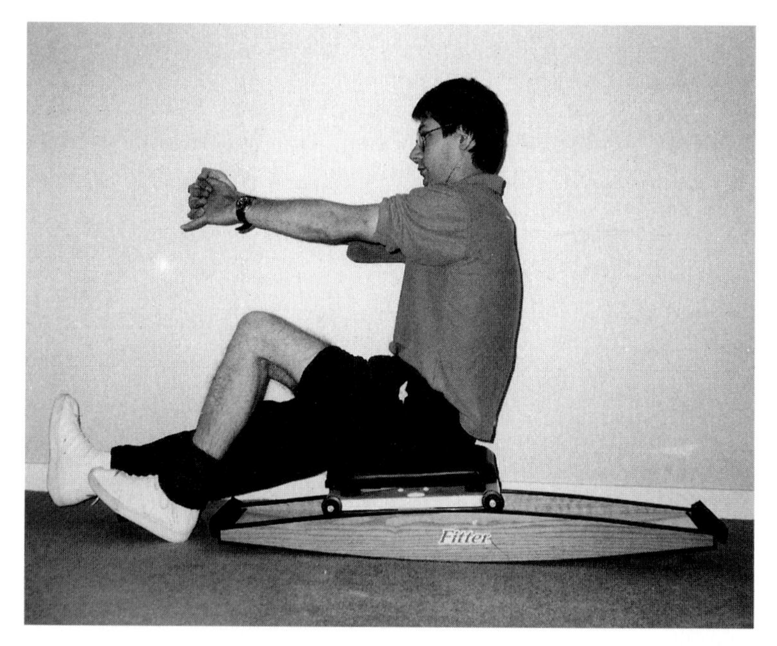

Fig. 121

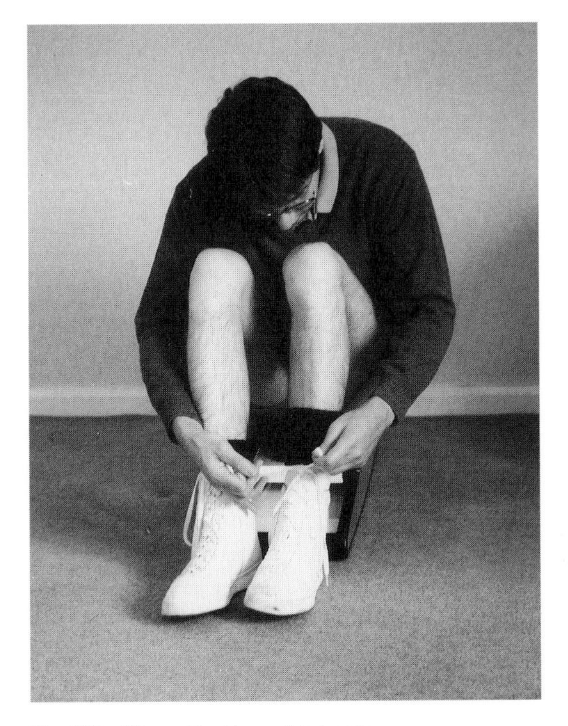

Fig. 122 The patient laces his boots.

APPENDIX

Some useful addresses:

Aircast
Aircast supply the Air-Stirrup Ankle Brace.
Order No. O2B/L Single or No. O2B/R Single; write for particulars.
Aircast, PO Box 709, Summit, New Jersey 07902–0709, USA.
UK: (Aircast) Orthopaedic Systems, Unit G22, Old Gate, St Michael, Cheshire WA8 8TL.

Arjo
Arjo Lift Walker 214141
Arjo Hospital Equipment is manufactured in Sweden by:
Arjo Hospital Equipment Ltd, Box 61, S-241, Eslöv, Sweden.
Arjo UK office: Arjo Hospital Equipment Ltd, SPD Building, Acre Road, Reading RG2 0SU.

Fitter
Fitter International Inc., 4515 1st St. S.E., Calgary, Alberta, Canada T2G 2L2.
Fitter UK. Marketed by:
Richard Haynes, The Coach House, Kirtlington, Oxford OX5 3HJ.

Flowpulse
Write for details of various Huntleigh models.
Huntleigh Technology plc, Health Care Division, 66 Bilton Way, Dallow Road, Luton, Beds LU1 1UU.

Follo
An alternative to the Arjo which also has adjustable height arm rests. Write for details.
The Walking Frame Eva. Follo, Industrier AS, PO Box 112, N-1430 As, Norway.

MJS Health Care Ltd
Intermittent compression; the 'Pulse Press 50' machine. This is an excellent, reasonably priced unit. Write for details.
MJS Health Care Ltd, Faldo Road, Barton-Le-Clay, Beds MK45 4RT.

URIAS
URIAS inflatable pressure splints. Write for details of distributors.
Splints include:
- URIAS Stroke rehabilitation splints
- URIAS MS therapy splints
- URIAS Child splints for paediatric conditions
- URIAS Baby splints for paediatric conditions.

Use URIAS splints to give support and control distribution of muscle tone.
Pharma-Plast, Medical Bag Division, Häarlev, DK 4652, Denmark.

Wolf turntable
Duffield Medical (Physiotherapy) Ltd, Newlands, Woodfall Lane, Nr. Quarndon, Derbyshire DE6 4L6 UK.

GLOSSARY

Active assisted movement Movement where the active action is assisted by an outside force.

Active movement Movement where no attempt is made to assist or resist the action.

Agnosia A perceptual disturbance giving difficulty in recognition.

Agonists Muscles which contract to produce movement (prime movers) against the weaker antagonists.

Agraphia Inability to express thoughts in writing.

Alexia Word blindness; loss of the ability to interpret the significance of the printed or written word, but without loss of visual power.

Anosognosia Failure to recognize the disability involving the forgotten half of the body; neglect or denial of ownership of the affected limbs.

Aphasia Inability to express thoughts in words; loss of the faculty of interchanging thought, where the intellect and will are unaffected.

Approximate To close together with pressure, as used when compression is applied through the articulating surface of a joint.

Apraxia A disturbance of visual–spatial relationships, or visual–spatial orientation, which leads to inability to manipulate objects effectively, or to carry a task through.

Articulation (As used here.) Enunciation of speech.

Assessment Informal but careful observation, leading to a decision on the state of the patient and the line of treatment to be followed.

Associated reactions These occur with all attempted movements and are released postural reactions deprived of voluntary control because of cortical damage. They produce a widespread increase in spasticity in the affected muscles if the limbs are not inhibited.

Astereognosis Failure to recognize familiar objects by their shape, size and texture when held in the hand with the eyes shut; tactile agnosia.

Body image The image in an individual's mind of his own body. Distortions of body image occur as a result of affective disorders, parietal lobe tumours or trauma, such as stroke.

Cognition Knowing or awareness, in the wider sense, including sensation, perception etc. Awareness, one of the three aspects of the mind, the others being affection (feeling or emotion), and conation (willing or desiring). They work as a whole but with cognitive disturbance one may dominate.

Cross-facilitation Working with the sound side of the body across the midline to the affected side to initiate bilateral activity.

Distal Furthest from the head or source.

Dysarthria A disorder of speech which includes difficulty in articulation due to motor defect in the muscles of lips, tongue, palate and throat.

Dysgraphia Difficulty in writing.

Dyslexia Difficulty in reading.

Dysphasia A disorder of language which may, or may not, include difficulty in comprehension. More usually, comprehension remains intact.

Equilibrium Balance; state of even balance; a state in which opposing forces or tendencies neutralize each other.

Equilibrium responses Responses which must include shifts in muscle tone and which make it possible for the body to equilibriate, or to balance or counterpoise, against any alterative situation caused by changes of position or environment.

Facilitate To make easy or easier.

Golgi tendon organs These are proprioceptors which lie at musculotendinous junctions. They are receptive to sustained stretch and are known to have an inhibitory influence on motoneurone pools of their own muscle supply; an autogenic effect.

Hemianopia Blindness in one half of the visual field of one or both eyes.

Hypertonia Excessive or more than normal tone.

Hypotonia A lack of, or less than normal, tone.

Ideation The process concerned with the highest function of awareness, the formation of ideas. It includes thought, intellect and memory.

Ideomotor Mental energy, in the form of ideas, producing automatic movement of muscles.

Ideopraxist One who is impelled to carry out an idea.

Infarct Area of tissue affected when the end artery supplying it is occluded, e.g. in the heart.

Irradiation Muscle activity which takes place when a strong muscle group acts against resistance to give an overflow of activity (or irradiation) into other parts of the body.

Jargon Confused talk.

Kinaesthesia Sense of movement or of muscular effort; perception of movement. (*Adj.* kinaesthetic.)

Muscle tone A state of slight tension of muscle fibres, when not in use, which enables them to respond more swiftly to a stimulus.

Neurone The structural unit of the nervous system comprising fibres (dendrites) which carry impulses to the nerve cell; the nerve itself, and the fibres (axons) which carry impulses from the cell. In the lower motor neurone the cell is in the spinal cord and the axon passes to skeletal muscle. In the upper motor neurone the cell is in the cerebral cortex and the axon passes down the spinal cord to arborize with a lower motor neurone.

Paraphasia A form of aphasia in which one word is substituted for another.

Parietal lobe The lobe of the brain which contains the sensory area.

Perception Act or power of perceiving; discernment; apprehension of any modification of consciousness; the combining of sensations into a recognition of an object.

Perseveration Meaningless repetition of an utterance (or an action, as in drawing); tendency to experience difficulty in leaving one thought for another.

Phonation Production of vocal sound.

PNF Proprioceptive neuromuscular facilitation. Method used to facilitate a response from the neuromuscular mechanism through stimulation of the proprioceptors.

Positioning Placing in the optimum position to allow for, and to promote, recovery.

Primitive movement Movement which is entirely reflex in character, fundamental, belonging to the beginning.

Prognosis Forecast, especially of the course of a disease.

Proprioceptive (*Adj.*) Pertaining to, or made active by, stimuli arising from movement in the tissues.

Proprioceptive sense The sense of muscular position, or of muscle and joint position.

Proprioceptor A sensory nerve ending receptive of sensory stimuli.

Protract To draw forward, or lengthen.

Proximal Nearest to the head or source.

Recovery pattern The pattern of movement which inhibits dominating reflexes in the stroke patient to allow for, and to promote, recovery. This must also include resting positions: positions in which the body is placed to allow for optimum recovery while at rest.

Rehabilitation Obtaining the maximum degree of physical and psychological independence after disability by means of a carefully planned physical programme which should be presented to the patient with cheerful optimism, an optimistic approach being a necessary part of successful rehabilitation.

Resistance Opposition.

Resisted movement Movement where resistance is given to gain a greater response, or to strengthen the action.

Retract To draw back or shorten.

Servo mechanism A mechanism serving automatically to control the working of another mechanism.

Spasm A violent involuntary muscular contraction; a state of continuous muscular contraction as opposed to intermittent contraction.

Spasticity In stroke, spasticity results because of the missing inhibitory influence from the brain which controls the normal balance of muscle tone to allow for reciprocal innervation of antagonistic pairs of muscles.

Spatial orientation Awareness of body position in relation to space.

Stable (As used here.) Able to recover equilibrium after being slightly displaced; not easily thrown off balance.

Stereognosis The recognition of familiar objects by their shape, size and texture when held in the hand with the eyes closed.

Stimulus An action, influence or agency that produces a response in a living organism.

Synapse The point of communication between two adjacent neurones.

Synergists Muscles which contract and relax in conjunction with prime movers crossing more than one point. NB: the synergic pattern of tonic contraction, therefore, results from hypertonic, or excessive, muscle tone leading to muscle contraction which follows the pattern of synergists.

Visual agnosia Failure to interpret what is seen. This type of 'blindness' usually clears up more slowly than hemianopia.

INDEX

Page numbers in bold refer to illustrations.

A

B

C

D

E

F

G

H

Q

R

S

T

V

W